P9-CFA-024

CHRIS JOHNSON'S

on target living™
NUTRITION
the power of feeling your best

Written by Chris Johnson

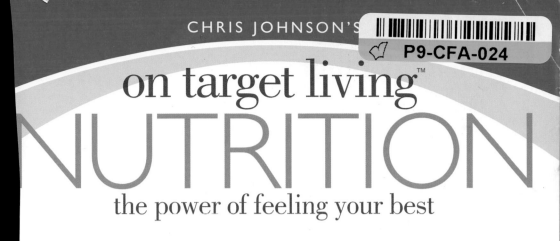

Design by CiesaDesign

Published by

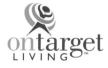

on target
LIVING™

ISBN 978-0-9727281-4-0
On Target Living, Int'l
Haslett, Michigan

table of contents

Acknowledgments/Dedication.. 6

Foreword... 7

Introduction: The Power of Feeling Your Best.............................. 9
   Diets don't work.. 10

SECTION 1: CHANGING YOUR LIFE 11

Chapter 1: We've Been Led Astray.. 12
   Why is our health at risk?.. 12
   Help has arrived 14
   The bottom line.. 14

Chapter 2: Why Diets Don't Work.. 16
   Scenario 1: Exchange/low-calorie diet.. 17
   Scenario 2: Low-fat, low-protein, high-carbohydrate diet............. 18
   Scenario 3: High-protein, high-fat, low-carbohydrate diet............. 19
   The 80/20 rule.. 21
   The bottom line.. 22

Chapter 3: Old Thinking—New Thinking....................................... 23
   Old Thinking: Skip meals to lose weight.. 23
   New Thinking: Eat small meals frequently..................................... 24
   Old Thinking: Cut calories to lose weight...................................... 25
   New Thinking: All calories are not created
   equal—quality counts.. 26
   Old Thinking: Eliminate fat from the diet....................................... 27
   New Thinking: Cut unhealthy fats and incorporate healthy fats..... 27
   Old Thinking: Eat anything and take supplements.......................... 27
   New Thinking: Focus on high-quality foods first............................ 28
   Summary of old and new thinking:... 29

Chapter 4: Healthy Cells Are Happy Cells.................................... 30
   The cell membrane... 31
   Mitochondria.. 32
   Nucleus of the cell... 33
   The bottom line.. 33

Chapter 5: Alkaline/Acid: Balancing the Body's pH.................... 34
   How do an acid-forming diet and high levels of stress
   lead to all of these health problems?.. 35
   What causes acid and alkaline to become unbalanced?................. 38
   What can I do to balance my acid and alkaline levels?................... 39
   The bottom line.. 41

Chapter 6: Going Organic.. 43
   What does "organic" mean?... 43
   How do you know it's organic?.. 43
   How much does it cost?.. 44
   The bottom line.. 45

Chapter 7: Laying the Foundation 46
Maslow's Hierarchy of Human Needs 46
The three building blocks of your foundation 47
The bottom line 51
Chapter 8: Let Food Be Your Medicine 53
Bonnie's journey 54
Medications can help 56
The bottom line 57
Chapter 9: Aim for the Food Target 59
USDA's Food Guidance—MyPyramid 59
On Target Living Nutrition: Food Target 61

SECTION 2:
THE CORE OF ON TARGET LIVING NUTRITION 63

Chapter 10: Fuel Your Body with Carbohydrates 66
Are carbohydrates healthy or unhealthy? 66
Fiber 68
Types of carbohydrates 71
The carbohydrate continuum 71
Carbohydrate chemistry 71
The glycemic index 73
Why do we crave carbohydrates? 75
The lowdown on sweet stuff 77
How many carbohydrates should you eat each day? 79
The bottom line 80
Chapter 11: Build Your Body with Protein 81
What is protein? 81
Benefits of protein 82
What kinds of protein should you eat? 83
The protein continuum 92
The bottom line 94
Chapter 12: Heal Your Body with Fats 95
Medical research supporting healthy fats 96
Where have we gone wrong? 97
Why is eating healthy fats so essential to optimal performance
and good health? 99
The categories of fats 100
Improving the quality of fat in your diet 115
The bottom line 116
Chapter 13: Check Your Fluids 119
Soda pop 119
Coffee 120
Tea 120
Milk 121

Juice.. 122
Sports drinks... 122
Energy drinks 124
Alcohol.. 124
Water: Your body's drink of choice 124
The bottom line.. 127

Chapter 14: The Key to Healthy Bones.......................... 128
What weakens bones?.. 129
What can you do to keep your bones healthy?......... 130
The bottom line.. 132

Chapter 15: What Should You Feed Your Kids?............ 133
Tips to get started.. 134
The bottom line.. 136

SECTION 3: STEPS TO SUCCESS................................. 137

Chapter 16: Putting It All Together................................. 138
Making the decision to change..................................... 138
What do you want to change? 139
Why do you want to change? 139
Plan to succeed and succeed with a plan.................. 139
The bottom line.. 143

Chapter 17: Write It Down.. 144
How to use the daily food log...................................... 145
The bottom line.. 145

Chapter 18: How to Read a Label................................... 147
How long is the ingredient list? 147
Do you recognize all the words in the ingredient list?....... 148
What is the serving size? 148
What kind of fat?.. 149
What type of sweetener? 150
What is the balance of carbohydrate, protein, and fat?....... 151
How was the food or beverage grown or processed?....... 152
The bottom line.. 152

Chapter 19: Shopping 101 153
The bottom line.. 155

Chapter 20: The Three-Hour Rule.................................. 156
The bottom line.. 157

Chapter 21: It's Quality, Quality, Quality 158
Incremental changes.. 158
Quantity—calories do count!....................................... 162
Quick-pick food list.. 166
The bottom line.. 168

Chapter 22: Balancing the "Big Three" 169
  Breakfast 170
  Lunch 171
  Dinner 172
  Snacks 173
  The bottom line 174

Chapter 23: Mindful Eating 175
  Increase your awareness 177
  Build your mindful eating action plan 178
  References 182
  The bottom line 183

Chapter 24: Healthy Eating on the Run 184
  Out-of-town travel 184
  Eating out 185
  The bottom line 187

Chapter 25: Make It Yours 188

Chapter 26: Exercise: The Fountain of Youth 192
  The bionic woman 192
  Why don't we exercise? 193
  Exercise and weight loss 198
  Posture alignment 199
  Getting started: How much exercise is enough? 200
  Equipment needs 210
  Sample exercise programs 211
  Frequently asked exercise questions 211
  Exercise considerations 214
  The bottom line 214

Chapter 27: Starting at Zero 215

Chapter 28: Taking It to the Next Level 219
  Taking-it-to-the-next-level plan 220

Chapter 29: You Can Do It! 223
  Final tips for success 223
  Enjoy the journey 226

APPENDICES 227
Appendix A: On Target Living Recipes 227
Appendix B: On Target Living Exercises 246
Appendix C: On Target Living Daily Logs 287

Index 291

acknowledgments/dedication

There are so many people who were instrumental in the development and completion of this book. I'd like to begin by thanking a few of my college professors: Dr. Louis Junker, Dr. Wayne Van Huss, Dr. William Heusner, and Dr. Kwok Ho. Thank you for sharing your passion and vision and opening my eyes to a life's work in health and fitness.

To my personal training clients who I have learned from, been supported by, and inspired me every step of the way.

To Lauren Ciesa, Michael Sundermann, Gerna Rubenstein, and Sandy Clark at CiesaDesign for your hard work, patience, guidance, creativity, and vision in putting this book together.

To my colleagues who have helped guide, inspire and keep the bar raised high. Your passion and energy for helping people are what life is all about.

To Al Arens, my mentor, for your guidance and friendship over the years.

Thanks to all my wonderful friends and family who have supported me and this project wholeheartedly.

To Bonnie Klinger—your transformation and spirit will change many lives;, it has changed my life.

To my faithful readers and followers, whose letters, emails, and testimonials have motivated me to expand my vision in helping people live healthier lives.

Last but not least, to my wife, Paula, and my kids, Kristen and Matt, for all your love and support.

Thanks.

CJ

foreword

How does one express his gratitude to someone who has helped him to achieve his goals, gain confidence to overcome physical and mental barriers to strive for better health, and help develop balance and symmetry in lifestyle, eating habits, body shape, and posture?

One would expect a cardiothoracic surgeon to have no problem attaining and maintaining the above-mentioned basic tenets of life, without difficulty, as if by second nature. Not necessarily. Let me explain!

I was brought up in Kampala, the capital city of Uganda, a small nation in the middle of Africa. My parents, both of whom were doctors, always pushed us to do our best—particularly in terms of our education—and helped me to pursue and achieve my career goals in the face of all kinds of difficulties.

After completing high school in Kampala, which in those days was in great political turmoil, I went to Bombay, India, to complete my medical degree. It was soon after that that my parents were forced to flee Uganda due to the regime of Idi Amin. My parents then immigrated to England after a short stay in India. I joined my family in England upon completing a surgical residency in Bombay, eager to pursue my dream of becoming a heart surgeon, inspired by Dr. Christian Barnard, who is responsible for putting Africa on the medical map by performing the first human heart transplant in the world.

Not satisfied with the support and opportunity afforded in England, I immigrated to the United States after a grueling, six-year surgical residency, which I had to repeat to become eligible to practice heart and lung surgery in this country. Finally, after having completed almost sixteen years of surgical residencies on three different continents, I settled in Lansing and have worked incessantly to establish myself in the practice of my chosen profession.

It was during these years that I ignored my personal health and allowed the vagaries of external forces to dictate my physical shape to the extent that, at six feet, I weighed over 250 pounds and did not have the stamina to carry out even moderate exertion. In addition, I used to get severe backaches and could not walk without becoming winded. Furthermore, I contracted tuberculosis during a visit abroad and almost died. God, however, had more in mind for me, and I gratefully recovered from the disease.

At this point I decided I should take better care of myself. But how? I tried a number of dietary regimens, including Atkins, South Beach, periods of starvation, etc., without any success. I also took up exercise, with the help of a number of trainers, but was not able to sustain my practice for long and lumbered back into my old habits of working hard, starving myself the entire day, followed by eating irresponsibly at night. This pattern, which lasted for about four to five years, did not result in any improvement. In addition, I became so frustrated I lost all faith in my ability to lose weight.

It was at this juncture in my life that I recognized I needed assistance and called Chris, whom I had known for some time. From the beginning, Chris seemed to be someone who knew not only how to help one achieve one's goals, but also maintain them. What impressed me most about Chris was his philosophy, which was all about balance, perseverance, and focus on fundamentals. This approach permeates not only Chris's exercise training regimen, but also his weight-loss regimen, as is evident in the book *On Target Living Nutrition*. In this particular book, Chris talks at length about the balance between carbohydrates, fats, and proteins, and the need to assimilate good- versus poor-quality food. Chris also emphasizes the need for gradual, progressive weight loss rather than rapid and, even worse, unbalanced weight loss, as recommended by some popular regimens. This same philosophy is evident in his exercise program, as Chris has focused on improving my core muscle development.

One would expect to understand this concept naturally, but despite the fact that my mother used to constantly remind me to walk erect as a child, I could not do it for any length of time until Chris helped me to develop my core muscle strength. With this combined approach, Chris has helped me lose over thirty-five pounds in weight. I now walk erect, fulfilling my mother's wishes, and can run over a mile and a half without difficulty. This may not sound like much to some people, but for me it is quite an accomplishment, and something I could never do even in high school. More importantly, Chris has instilled the confidence in me to know I can accomplish the next phase of my goal, which is to continue to lose more weight and maintain it, while living a healthy life for a long time to come.

So, Chris, thank you very much for all you have done for me, and if my experience inspires someone else to take the path to strive for excellence in health and fitness, then I would be satisfied that the gratitude has been expressed to a small degree!

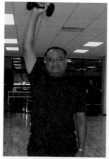

With much respect,

Divyakant B. Gandhi, M.D., FACS, FRCS
Attending Cardiothoracic Surgeon
Assistant Clinical Professor of Surgery
College of Human Medicine and College of Osteopathic Medicine
Michigan State University

introduction

THE POWER OF
FEELING YOUR BEST

Imagine feeling great, better than you have for a long time—maybe ever. Imagine having lots of energy, feeling strong with greater vitality. Can you remember the last time you felt that good? Have you *ever* felt that good? Feeling great, or not, is closely connected to your nutrition—how you nurture, nourish, and fuel your body.

> The future belongs to those who believe in the beauty of their dreams.
>
> —Eleanor Roosevelt

With *On Target Living Nutrition* you get a chance for a fresh start with food: how you think about it and what you do with it. It will open the door for you to understand why what you eat affects every aspect of your life. By using the simple tools in this book, you can quickly achieve optimal health and performance for your body and your life.

If you are overweight, you will lose weight following the *On Target Living Nutrition* principles. More importantly, though, you will gain the knowledge and the power to manage your weight for the rest of your life. The focus of *On Target Living Nutrition* is health and vitality, not just weight loss.

I believe most people have three goals when it comes to their nutritional program:

1. To maintain or improve their health
2. To feel good and have energy throughout the day
3. To control their weight.

With *On Target Living Nutrition*, **you can achieve all three.**

Start your journey by turning the page.
Here's to Your Health!

DIETS DON'T WORK

Many clients come to me as a last resort. They've tried countless diets, supplements, drinks, pills, and elixirs. The problem is that diets don't work. Experience has proven this. Not only do diets set up a destructive cycle of deprivation and indulgence, they have one fundamental flaw: A diet is a short-term "fix." By definition, diets end. Without a basic understanding of how food works in the body, once the diet is over the dieter hasn't learned how to manage situations that don't exactly fit the diet. They get bored. Counting and computing calories become tedious and unrealistic, so people stop doing it. Sooner or later, they end up right back where they started. Only it's worse because they feel as though they've failed; they feel hopeless. But there *is* hope. And it's easier than you think.

On Target Living Nutrition offers a completely different and far more powerful approach. Dieters lack options because they don't develop the knowledge they need to make healthy, reasonable choices with the intention of nourishing their bodies. *On Target Living Nutrition* gives you options because it gives you information and the understanding of what your body needs to perform. It gives you options with a vast array of delicious, satisfying foods, and the knowledge of how your body uses food for nourishment and fuel. Most importantly, *On Target Living Nutrition* gives you the power to take control of your choices based on knowledge, information, and understanding so you can feel great, all the time.

Simply—*On Target Living Nutrition* will give you the power to feel your best.

TAKE IT FROM ME...

I have prescribed On Target Living to hundreds of my patients for many reasons—diabetes, heart disease, high cholesterol, hypertension, obesity, fatigue, even fibromyalgia. On Target Living is a comprehensive approach to healthy eating and healthy living. Ninety-eight percent of the people who bought the On Target Living book said it had a positive impact on their lives and they would buy it again. As a doctor, I find it particularly noteworthy that the most recent nutritional recommendations for heart disease incorporate the same core concepts that Chris Johnson has taught for over fifteen years.

—Ralph Harvey, M.D.
Family Practice

changing your life

Chapter 1

WE'VE BEEN LED ASTRAY

Let's lay the cards on the table. Even with greater advances in medicine, more highly trained health professionals, more medications to choose from, and an overwhelming amount of information on the benefits of proper rest, nutrition, and exercise to help keep our bodies healthy, Americans are doing a lousy job when it comes to managing their health!

With all that we have learned, and all the resources at our disposal, this sad fact is true and, more importantly, getting worse! It is estimated that more than 150 million Americans now live with at least one chronic disease or disability. According to the Centers for Disease Control and Prevention, chronic illness accounts for more than three-quarters of all the money now spent on health care in the United States. Obesity has doubled since 1985. More than 15 million Americans have Type 2 diabetes. Over 20 percent of women over age fifty have thyroid problems. Acid reflux and irritable bowel syndrome are common, everyday problems for many adults. Poor bone health is evident in many young women, and *over one-third of our children are overweight.* The picture is not pretty, and we all need to get in the game of health.

> **Prevention is so much better than healing.**
>
> —Thomas Adams

WHY IS OUR HEALTH AT RISK?

Poor-quality food environment

The food environment in which we live has changed dramatically over the last thirty years. We now have greater access to large quantities of cheap, low-quality food. In the early 1980s we consumed approximately 3,100 calories per person, per day, in the United States. Today we are consuming more than 4,100 calories per person. As you can probably guess, we are not consuming more *whole foods,* such as fruits and vegetables, whole grains, high-quality proteins, and healthy fats. Whole foods are nutrient-dense and make your body healthy and help you perform at your best. Unfortunately, we are producing unhealthier, refined, nutrient-deficient junk food!

Everywhere you turn you see low-quality, cheap food—from airports, fast-food restaurants, gas stations, grocery stores, big box stores, schools, and vending machines.

We are a nation of convenience-food consumers. Convenience translates into highly processed, poor-quality food. As our lives speed up, so does the demand for convenient, fast, available food.

Food companies produce poor-quality food and beverages because we continue to buy them. What do I mean by poor-quality food and beverages? Take an orange for example. An orange is a whole food. It has only one ingredient. It has not been refined or processed, so it contains many vitamins, minerals, antioxidants, and fiber—ingredients that make the body healthy. What happens to an orange when it is highly processed or refined? Does it have the same healthy benefits as a whole orange? When an orange is processed into orange juice, it's

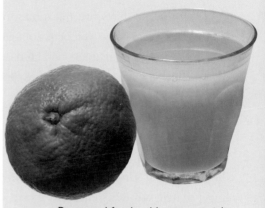

Processed foods add nonessential ingredients and take away essential ones.

still a good choice, but you lose the fiber you would get from eating the whole orange. Take the orange juice and further refine it into "orange drink." You now have a product that no longer resembles a whole orange.

As consumers become more educated about the benefits of eating higher-quality foods, the demand for higher-quality foods will increase. Until we begin to change our buying practices, companies will continue to produce poor-quality, nutritionally deficient foods.

Lack of physical activity

The time we spend being physically active continues to decline. Our kids seldom walk to school. They sit in the classroom, sit behind the computer, sit in front of video games, and sit watching television. Physical education classes have been cut from many of our school systems. Fewer than 25 percent of American adults exercise regularly.

Regular exercise has a host of wonderful benefits, but many people choose not to make time to move their bodies on a regular basis.

Poor information

Many different approaches to eating and physical activity are advocated through popular culture, the media, books, magazines, friends, and family, leaving the consumer in a state of flux and confusion. Even when we want to live healthier lives through better eating and exercise, it is difficult to know what information is accurate.

Pervasive dieting mentality

Over the last thirty-five years, hundreds of fad diets and trendy ways of eating have bombarded Americans. New books, magazines, testimonials, and infomercials bring the promise of instant weight loss and fitness. With each promise, it's easy to see why many of us will try any new diet that comes along if the claims are powerful enough.

HELP HAS ARRIVED

Okay, enough of the doom and gloom! I am a real believer in the "law of attraction": what you focus your attention on you will attract into your life. So let's focus on the good news! The human body is truly amazing in how it tries to heal itself. We all know that if you cut your hand it will start to heal itself in just a few days. If you struggle with your weight, have low energy or poor health, or would just like to feel better and perform at a higher level, help has arrived! I have seen tremendous life changes in many people during the two decades I have been in the health and fitness industry. I would like to help you as well.

THE BOTTOM LINE

1. Americans are in serious trouble when it comes to their eating habits and overall health.
2. Over 150 million Americans now live with at least one chronic disease or disability.
3. Over 60 percent of Americans are overweight and out of shape.
4. We are failing due to easy access to unhealthy food, lack of exercise, poor information, and a quick-fix dieting mentality.
5. The human body is truly amazing in its ability to heal itself if given the right ingredients.

TAKE IT FROM ME...

My name is Karen Griffin. I am thirty-four years old, married, and have two small children. In 1990, I was at a healthy 150 pounds. Fifteen years later, in January 2005, I was shocked to find myself weighing in at 232 pounds! In addition to the weight gain, I found myself becoming more and more exhausted, depressed, angry, with unstable blood glucose levels, frequent anxiety attacks, very low self-image, withdrawing from society, and medicating myself with more food. In addition, I had daily headaches and was taking a minimum of eight to ten pain relievers every day.

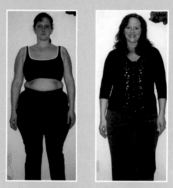

Karen Griffin, Paw Paw, Michigan

In February 2005, I went to the doctor for my depression and anxiety. The doctor wanted to put me on antidepressant medication and anti-anxiety medication, but never mentioned anything about me being seriously overweight. I left the doctor's office with the prescription orders in my hand, but never filled the orders. A few weeks later, I ran into an old friend who is one of the healthiest people I know and she gave me Chris Johnson's book to read.

Since I had been "dieting" for the last fifteen years, and read practically every weight-loss book out there, I was happy to read yet another book about dieting. I only read a few pages before I realized that it was not a diet book at all! I was intrigued, so I kept reading. I read the entire book in two days! I immediately began reading it again. The second time through, something started to "click" in my mind. For the first time in my life, I started to look at food from a nutritional value instead of a calorie/point value. Suddenly, my focus turned from trying to lose weight (at whatever cost) to making healthy food choices and feeling good from the inside out.

So many nutrition books go over the average reader's head. It was refreshing to read a book that I could understand. But after reading *On Target Living Nutrition* for the first time, I was overwhelmed by all of the information. Where should I start? What should I change first? So I did as the book suggested, and just started making small changes. I put the *Food Target* on my refrigerator and eliminated most items from the outer ring. Then I began eating six small meals a day—and immediately felt better! My blood glucose began to stabilize, I wasn't tired, I was happier, had fewer cravings, and—as an added bonus—I began to lose weight. I could not believe that I could eat every three hours and lose weight—and never be hungry! Wow! Where has this information been all of my life? Shortly after, I started really focusing on the quality of the six meals I was eating, started focusing on the inner rings of the *Food Target*. I added flaxseeds, fish oils, and many organic products. I also was very dedicated to drinking more water every day and added some cardiovascular and strength training to my life.

And here I am now, more than two years later. I have lost over forty pounds and continue to lose. But most importantly, I feel better than I have ever felt. I am a completely different person on the inside and outside. I am a better mother and wife. I am happy, full of energy, I actually like myself again, and no more anxiety, no blood glucose problems, and I haven't had a headache in almost a year! I never realized that the food I was putting in my body was a drug—until I stopped using that drug and "got clean." Since my friend shared Chris's book with me, I now feel like I have a responsibility to spread the good news and tell the world that there is hope. If I can do it, so can they. I just want everyone to have the opportunity to feel as good as I do—because I truly believe that reading this book saved not only my marriage, but my life.

Chapter 2
WHY DIETS DON'T WORK

Hundreds of new diet programs hit the market every year. The American population is obsessed with weight loss, spending *over $50 billion a year* on weight loss related products and services.

A few years ago there was a seminar in my hometown titled "How to Outsmart the Female Fat Cell." Over 350 women, along with a few men, showed up for this seminar! I wasn't the only one intrigued by this catchy title. I have to be honest with you, I was a little disappointed that I didn't come up with this title myself. The speaker did a nice job. She talked about the importance of controlling stress, eating healthy foods, and fitting regular exercise into each day. This was all great stuff, but it was not the magic secret people were hoping to hear.

I am asked on a daily basis to look at some new piece of exercise equipment, supplement, sports drink, or super food. People are looking for that special something that will help them lose weight. Look at all the infomercials on television today trying to get you to buy a particular weight-loss product.

> **Every problem has in it the seeds of its own solution.**
>
> —Norman Vincent Peale

A few years ago I was channel surfing and came across one of these infomercials. The product being sold was an "ice-cold water machine," a machine that would chill normal tap water to an extremely cold temperature. The selling point—drink this ice-cold water and your body will use additional calories to heat it. You will burn more calories and magically lose weight by just drinking this ice-cold water. That sounds pretty simple, drink water and lose weight! For three easy payments you too can have one of these fat-burning, ice-cold water machines in your house, and have the body you always dreamed about. *This stuff may sound convincing, but remember, there is no such thing as "the one thing."*

Making lifestyle changes can be difficult, especially if you are trying to make too many changes at once. If one of your goals is to lose weight, you need to understand a few fundamental principles about the science of weight loss. Without knowing these basic principles, dieters continue to search for a plan that is "right" for them.

Let's examine some of the most popular diets that capture people's attention with the promise of quick and painless weight loss. *Each of these diets lacks one or more principles for successful, healthy, long-term weight loss.*

SCENARIO 1: EXCHANGE/LOW-CALORIE DIET

The exchange/low-calorie diet is a relatively balanced eating program in which you make choices called "exchanges" within similar groups of foods. It is a portion-control diet plan that restricts calories by limiting the number and type of exchanges from each of the food groups. Dieters are sometimes encouraged to save their exchanges if they want to reward themselves with a certain type of disallowed food or splurge on a favorite food.

Lack of attention to the quality of foods is the main shortcoming of an exchange program. It is fairly well balanced with carbohydrates, proteins, and fats, though somewhat low on quality fats. An exchange program gives little consideration to the nutritional composition or quality of foods the dieter consumes. There's a big difference between the quality of extra-virgin olive oil and margarine, yet both count as a fat exchange. Wild Alaskan salmon and a fat-free hot dog count as equivalent protein exchanges. The salmon, however, provides the highest-quality nutrients for your cells. I tried this diet for a few days, but was running out of fat exchanges by noon!

Typical exchange diet menu	
Breakfast	cold cereal fruit skim milk toast with fat-free margarine coffee
Snack	low-fat breakfast bar
Lunch	low-calorie frozen entrée
Dinner	chicken breast steamed broccoli baked potato with nonfat sour cream
Snack	fat-free frozen yogurt

TAKE IT FROM ME...

I wish to compliment you on your outstanding On Target Living presentations to our associates. I cannot begin to tell you the enthusiasm you have created at Auto-Owners for people to begin a healthier lifestyle. I think the best compliment a speaker or writer can get is knowing that they made a difference to the people they touched. You have truly made an impact with the Auto-Owners team.

—Roger Looyenga, CEO, Auto-Owners Insurance Company (Fortune 500 Company)

SCENARIO 2: LOW-FAT, LOW-PROTEIN, HIGH-CARBOHYDRATE DIET

With the low-fat, low-protein, high-carbohydrate diet, fat is the villain! One fat gram contains nine calories, whereas carbohydrates and proteins have four calories per gram. This diet drastically reduces or eliminates dietary fat and replaces it with low-fat or no-fat products. It also severely restricts meat to control dietary fat. The diet allows water, coffee, and diet soda freely throughout the day and with meals. It discourages most snacking, though it allows some light snacking on vegetables. A typical daily menu for a high-carbohydrate, low-fat, low-protein dieter is shown.

Typical high-carbohydrate diet menu	
Breakfast	bagel cream cheese orange juice coffee
Snack	apple
Lunch	salad with vegetables fat-free raspberry vinaigrette dressing one piece whole-grain bread
Snack	two rice cakes two pieces hard candy
Dinner	pasta with marinara sauce salad with nonfat dressing two breadsticks
Snack	air-popped popcorn

Nutritionally, the composition of this diet overlooks quality proteins and healthy fats and overemphasizes carbohydrates. The intent of the diet is to restrict calories by reducing dietary fat in the hope that there will be a corresponding reduction in body fat. The old "you-are-what-you-eat" thinking. The problem is that restriction of dietary fat doesn't directly translate to a reduction in body fat. Body fat reduction is a complex physiological process that involves a number of factors. The human body needs a certain amount of high-quality fat every day. Eliminating fat from the diet is extremely risky to overall health and makes the diet difficult to maintain for any length of time. This low-fat, low-protein, high-carbohydrate diet will create not only a state of low energy, but a feeling of constant hunger, hormonal imbalance, and perhaps an increase in body fat as a result. The reasons for the consequences of this diet plan will be clear as you read on and gain a better understanding of nutrition.

SCENARIO 3: HIGH-PROTEIN, HIGH-FAT, LOW-CARBOHYDRATE DIET

In this diet, carbohydrates are the enemy. The idea is that by severely restricting carbohydrates, the body will burn protein and fat, thereby reducing body fat. Many find this diet easy to follow because of the liberal fat and protein allowances. The only foods that are limited are those high in carbohydrates. On this diet you can eat bacon, mayonnaise, prime rib, sausage, gravy— almost anything that doesn't seem like it belongs on a diet. What you *don't* eat are fruits, some vegetables, and whole grains. This diet also lacks an emphasis on quality fats and proteins. A typical menu may look like the one at the right.

Typical high-protein diet menu	
Breakfast	two eggs four strips bacon coffee
Snack	two slices cheese

Lunch	hamburger (no bun)
	  with cheese
	lettuce salad with ranch
	  dressing

Snack	chicken salad with mayonnaise
Dinner	sirloin steak lettuce salad with ranch dressing
Snack	cheddar cheese

If you severely restrict the carbohydrates in your diet (fruits, vegetables, legumes, whole grains, starches), you will burn fat and protein for energy, thereby eating up all that unwanted body fat that you desperately want to get rid of. The promise: limit carbohydrates, burn up more fat. Sounds great! However, there is more to this story.

One reason for the continued popularity of the high-protein, high-fat, low-carbohydrate diet is that the initial weight loss is quick. Losing four to seven pounds in the first week on this diet is common. However, the initial weight loss is primarily due to a loss in water and stored muscle glycogen. When carbohydrates are restricted in your diet, the body looks to its carbohydrate reserves (glycogen) for fuel. Each gram of glycogen binds with four grams of water. The human body only holds approximately 500 grams of glycogen. Within just a few days of restricted carbohydrate intake, your carbohydrate reserves will be depleted, leading to quick weight loss in the form of glycogen and water. As you add carbohydrates back into your diet your glycogen will act like a sponge and absorb water, leading to weight gain.

The major drawback of this diet is the severe damage it can do to your health. If you restrict carbohydrate intake, you deny your body important vitamins, minerals, phytochemicals, antioxidants, fiber, and food for the brain. The human brain needs approximately 400 calories per day to function properly. Carbohydrate is the only source of fuel that the brain can use for energy. Once the body has used up its carbohydrate reserves (glycogen), it begins to break down fat and protein for energy. You may be thinking, "what is wrong with using stored body fat as energy?" Well, without carbohydrates, the body begins to convert fat into energy, but the by-product of this conversion is an abnormal biochemical called *ketone bodies*. The body tries to rid itself of these highly acidic ketone bodies through increased urination and respiration. When fat cells go through this abnormal process to supply energy to the brain, *future fat cells can become up to ten times more efficient in storing fat.*

One of the most detrimental side effects of this high-protein, high-fat, low-carbohydrate diet is the *pH* changes that begin to occur throughout the body. Adding extra protein and thus limiting your carbohydrate intake causes your body to become too *acidic.* As your body becomes acidic, minerals are leached out of the body to buffer the high acid levels. Along with high acid levels, increased levels of oxidation occur through-out the body due to the lack of fruits and vegetables. Colorful fruits and vegetables contain a wide array of vitamins, minerals, and antioxidants. When these foods are not consumed on a daily basis, oxidation increases, leading to dry skin, brittle hair, and most of all, poor health! (More will be said on pH balance in Chapter 5.)

All things considered, this type of diet represents a serious risk to overall health and well-being. While it may deliver on the short-term promise of rapid weight loss, it can't deliver long-term good health.

TAKE IT FROM ME...

As an executive coach, I'm always recommending Chris's books and materials to my clients who want to improve their health and increase their energy. His information is easy to understand and implement immediately. So many of my clients tape the *Food Target* on their refrigerators! As I work with my clients on expanding their leadership capabilities, attention to health goes hand-in-hand with creating great leaders.

On a personal note, I have benefited greatly from working with Chris as a trainer and also hearing him many times as a keynote speaker. He is such a dynamic and engaging speaker! Each time I hear Chris speak about On Target Living, I add one more "healthy" choice to my shopping cart. In addition, Chris has helped me to work in exercise in my busy life juggling time between my business, my home, and motherhood.

—Susan Combs, Executive Coach

THE 80/20 RULE

The next time you are thinking about going on a diet, consider these questions: "Is this program something I can sustain? Can I really live on 1,200 calories per day? No fruit? Little fat? Or only raw foods?" Most of us at one time or another may have tried some type of diet only to abandon the mission after a specified period of time or specific result, ultimately returning to our old way of eating. A better option is to follow what I call the "80/20 rule."

The 80/20 rule is a healthy eating plan that you can follow for the rest of your life. Eighty percent of the time you eat in a healthy way. Most of your food choices fall in the green areas of the *Food Target*. The other 20 percent of the time you allow yourself to enjoy foods or beverages that may be outside the green area. When you vow to give up eating a certain food you like, you end up focusing on that food even more. You feel deprived.

Let's say you give up ice cream for good. You may then resent it whenever someone else has ice cream, and you will ultimately abandon your pledge. The point with the 80/20 rule is you can have ice cream 20 percent of the time if you want. Too many restrictions make most people want the forbidden foods even more.

One of my personal training clients, Stephanie Maat, gave me the idea of the 80/20 rule. Stephanie originally came to see me about improving her cholesterol and blood chemistry numbers, but also wanted to lose weight. After eight weeks of following the *On Target Living Nutrition* plan, she was feeling frustrated that she had not lost weight. She explained that she was eating many high-quality foods from the center of the *Food Target*, but the scale was not budging. I asked Stephanie to consider how many days in each month she ate in a healthy way. She thought about it for a few minutes and I think her answer surprised her. She said she ate healthy approximately fifteen days a month! As soon as she said fifteen days a month, she knew what the problem was. She was following the 50/50 rule! She was not gaining weight, but she was not losing either. Her curiosity was piqued and she asked what it would take for her to lose weight. I told her to do exactly what she had been doing on her better days, but do it more frequently. Stephanie came up with the 80/20 rule. In a one-month period she would eat healthy (only green areas of the *Food Target*) for twenty-four days and treat herself only six days of the month. Three months later Stephanie had lost twenty-five pounds and her blood chemistry had greatly improved without medications. Stephanie says she feels fantastic and has found a plan that she can live with the rest of her life.

Your goal with *On Target Living Nutrition* is to make small changes and slowly develop an eating plan that you can enjoy and sustain.

THE BOTTOM LINE

1. Americans are obsessed with weight loss, spending over $50 billion a year on weight loss–related products and services.
2. Lack of attention to the quality of foods is the main challenge of an exchange diet program.
3. Eliminating healthy fat from the diet by following a high-carbohydrate, low-fat program is extremely risky to overall health and is very difficult to sustain.
4. A high-protein, high-fat, low-carbohydrate diet denies the body important vitamins, minerals, phytochemicals, antioxidants, fiber, and food for the brain.
5. Most conventional diets address only weight loss and downplay or ignore optimal health and energy.
6. The 80/20 rule is a great tool in developing an eating plan that you can sustain and live with.

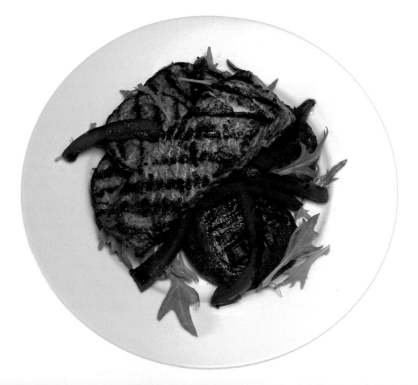

Chapter 3

OLD THINKING— NEW THINKING

OLD THINKING: Skip meals to lose weight

A favorite trick of practiced dieters is to skip meals to lose weight. Many dieters starve themselves all day and eat only an evening meal. Let's look at the value of this technique by acquainting ourselves with sumo wrestlers, who are experts at gaining weight. The sumos have learned that it's not just what you eat, but also how and when you eat, and what you do after eating that make you gain weight. To gain weight, the sumos gorge. They

> ## The biggest temptation is... to settle for too little.
> —Thomas Menton

eat one or two meals of 3,500 to 4,500 calories each day. Immediately after eating, they take a two- to three-hour nap.

As an example, one budding sumo wrestler initially weighing in at 350 pounds ate 6,000 calories a day spread over three meals. His typical calorie intake was 2,000 calories at breakfast, 2,500 at lunch, and 1,500 at dinner. He was considered a "lightweight."

In order to gain weight, he changed the patterns of his meals. After eighteen months, he had gained almost 230 pounds while cutting his caloric intake by 2,000 calories a day. How did he do it? He simply adopted the lifestyle of established sumo wrestlers. He changed his eating frequency yet lowered his quantity. Instead of three meals a day, he reduced it to one meal a day. Instead of consuming 6,000 calories a day, he ate 4,000 calories in that one daily meal. Additionally, he went to sleep immediately after eating.

4,000 calories × one meal/day + nap = 230 pound weight gain in 18 months

How is it possible to reduce the total calories consumed and the frequency of meals, yet still gain weight? It is possible because of two processes the body uses to protect itself from starvation.

First, your body protects itself from skipped meals by secreting the enzyme *lipoprotein lipase*. Lipoprotein lipase is the key enzyme that stores fat to protect the body from starvation. When you decrease the frequency of your meals or snacks, your lipoprotein lipase enzymes become more sensitive to storing calories. As the frequency of

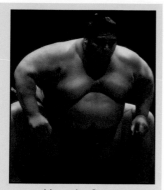

How the Sumo Gained Weight
- Decreased his frequency of eating
- Increased the quantity of the meal
- Went to sleep immediately after eating

your meals decreases, your lipoprotein lipase enzymes begin to work overtime in an effort to store extra calories as fat throughout your body.

Second, after eating, the body's blood glucose level rises, initiating a release of the hormone insulin. Insulin opens cells to use nutrients. Once the cells' needs are met, the remainder of the nutrients is stored as body fat. The increase in insulin levels leads to an increase in body fat stores as well as greater insulin resistance.

By the way, many sumo wrestlers develop Type 2 diabetes by the age of thirty and many die in their late forties.

NEW THINKING:
Eat small meals frequently

The adage of three square meals a day belongs in the old-thinking category. New thinking balances your total calories evenly throughout the day in five to six small meals of roughly equal proportion.

Look closely at the difference in how these calories are consumed, and think back to the sumo wrestlers and their gorging habits. Our old thinking would have us skip one or more meals, avoid snacking, and then gorge at one meal, usually dinner. We're so hungry by then that we eat anything we can put our hands on—candy, crackers, chips, cookies—and then eat dinner on top of that.

Meal	Old Thinking	New Thinking
breakfast	none	400 calories
snack	none	250 calories
lunch	500 calories	400 calories
snack	none	250 calories
dinner	1,500 calories	550 calories
snack	none	150 calories
total	2,000	2,000

New thinking spaces meals evenly throughout the day, including light snacks at mid-morning, mid-afternoon, and evening. By increasing the frequency of your eating, you will increase your metabolic rate, maintain a steadier blood glucose level, and reduce your chances of overeating at a given meal. Plus, you will not be hungry during the day. Other benefits of spacing out your meals will be better mental focus all day (avoiding the typical 3:00 p.m. slump that often leads to binge eating at dinner) and having a balanced sense of well-being and energy throughout the day and evening. *Bottom line:* You will just plain feel better and have a smaller waistline.

OLD THINKING: Cut calories to lose weight

Many people lose weight by reducing calories, only to gain back the weight and then some. Reducing the number of calories consumed daily is usually the first thing people do when they want to lose weight. Unfortunately, this is the wrong choice.

One fundamental rule for long-term control of body fat is to maintain or increase lean muscle tissue. If you lose weight by restricting calories, a large percentage of your weight loss is often due to a loss of lean muscle tissue. As your lean muscle decreases, your body's ability to burn calories at rest (resting metabolic rate) decreases. Each pound of lean muscle tissue burns 60 to 70 percent more calories at rest than each pound of fat. For every pound of fat that you replace with muscle, your body burns more calories and your resting metabolic rate increases. That is why regular exercise is critical for long-term control of body fat.

A common weight-loss approach is to determine the number of calories required to maintain your current weight and reduce the number of calories consumed accordingly. For example, if your body needs 2,000 calories per day to maintain your current weight, the theory is that by cutting back to 1,500 calories per day, you should lose one pound per week (7 days × 500 calorie deficit per day = 3,500 calories = one pound of fat loss). Adding exercise to the plan is a bonus and calories burned through exercise should contribute to further weight loss. This approach seems pretty simple. Eat less, exercise more, and watch the weight fall off. Unfortunately, it's not that simple.

The number of calories a person needs each day depends on many variables, including activity level, frequency of meals, food quality, quantity of food at each meal, lean muscle tissue, food combinations, genetic factors, and stress levels. It is possible to cut calories and still gain body fat. The amount of food, measured by number of calories you eat each

Imagine purchasing a $5 million racehorse and then feeding it low-quality foods. Worse, feeding it poor foods only once or twice a day, on schedule, regardless of whether it was hungry, had worked hard, or how it was expected to perform. Add inadequate rest, not enough water, and limited or no exercise to the dietary neglect and you have a racehorse with little or no chance of winning.

day, is one factor in the weight-loss equation, but it is not the best or only factor to attain weight loss or good health.

With *On Target Living Nutrition,* you will learn that calories are important, but the quality of food you eat, the combination of fat, protein, and carbohydrate, along with frequency of eating, have equal importance in the weight-loss and good health formula.

NEW THINKING: All calories are not created equal—quality counts

The old thinking that focuses on counting and restricting calories treats all calories as equal. A calorie-restriction program treats calories from bad fats and refined sugars the same as it does calories from high-quality protein, good fats, and unrefined carbohydrates, such as fruits and vegetables.

How are your cells affected in these two meals?	
one piece chocolate cake	one organic chicken breast one cup baked broccoli with extra-virgin olive oil

Chocolate cake	Chicken/broccoli/extra-virgin olive oil
Huge spike in blood glucose leading to a drop in energy	Small spike in blood glucose leading to sustained energy
Low energy, lethargic thought process, irritability, anxiety	Great energy, clear thought process, elevated mood
Spike in insulin, increased fat storage, and more food cravings, adding to the waistline	Small release of insulin, less fat storage, reduced food cravings, leading to a lean, fit body
Poorly balanced, low in vitamins and minerals, high in poor fats and refined sugars, leading to poor health	Well-balanced, high in vitamins, minerals, fiber, and high-quality fats, leading to hormonal balance and optimal health

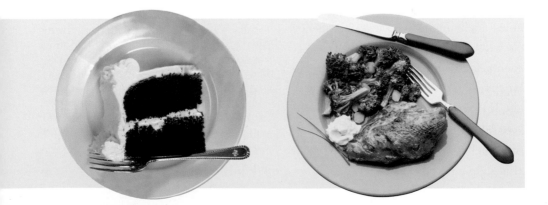

Consider how each meal impacts your energy, mood, health, and waistline during the three to four hours after you consume it. The quality of the foods you eat has an immense effect on your performance, health, and well-being.

OLD THINKING: Eliminate fat from the diet

Most people think that fats make you fat and unhealthy. Many diet programs advise reducing or eliminating all fats from the diet. The thinking is that reducing fats is an effective way to reduce the total calories that a person eats and that all fats cause diseases such as heart disease, high cholesterol, high blood pressure, obesity, cancer, and Type 2 diabetes.

NEW THINKING: Cut unhealthy fats and incorporate healthy fats

As with calories, not all fats are created equal. It is true that there is a predominance of fat in the typical American diet that contributes to poor health and disease. These unhealthy fats include trans-fatty acids (partially hydrogenated oils), refined saturated fats, and refined omega-6 fats. These are fats to avoid in your diet.

It is also true that *some* fats are essential for optimal health, performance, and weight control. These fats include some unrefined saturated fats, monounsaturated fats, and unrefined polyunsaturated fats. Refer to Chapter 12 for a thorough discussion of all the fats. The benefits of healthy fats include:
- Insulation of the body—providing thermoregulation
- Production of energy
- Protection of the body's major organs
- Maintenance of cell membrane structures
- Transportation of fat-soluble vitamins
- Hormonal balance

OLD THINKING: Eat anything and take supplements

People interested in changing their health and eating habits have dramatically increased their use of dietary supplements. Unfortunately, much of this increase stems from the pursuit of a "magic pill" to take the place of a more sensible and successful approach. The marketing of such products is very convincing. "Eat whatever you want with no exercise." "Take this supplement and watch fat melt away." "Take this supplement before bedtime and wake up thinner." These products, at best, produce only short-term results and, at worst, can be dangerous. Can you take that magic pill for the rest of your life? There is no such thing as a magic pill.

NEW THINKING: Focus on high-quality foods first

Supplements have their place and can be beneficial—or essential—for many people. However, supplements are not the place to start with your nutrition program. *On Target Living Nutrition* begins with the heavyweights, the macronutrients: carbohydrates (CHO), proteins (PRO), and fats (FAT). These are the foundation of what we consume daily and have the largest impact on our overall health and well-being. Consuming whole foods containing carbohydrates, proteins, and fats will have a much greater impact on your health than any supplement ever could.

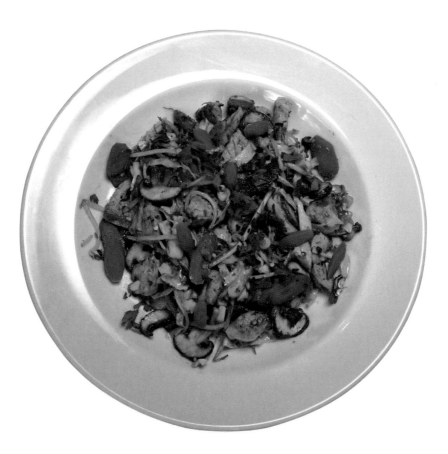

SUMMARY of old and new thinking

My intent with this book is to help you focus on new ways of thinking and learn how to incorporate new choices based on that thinking into your daily life for improved health and vitality. Here's a quick reminder of the differences between old and new thinking:

Old Thinking	New Thinking
Skip meals to lose weight	Eat small meals frequently
Cut calories to lose weight	All calories are not created equal
Eliminate fat from the diet	Improve the quality of your fats
Eat anything and take supplements	Eat quality foods first

TAKE IT FROM ME...

About six months ago during a routine physical and after numerous blood tests I was diagnosed with a life-threatening liver disease. My family doctor, along with a well-known specialist, prescribed a series of treatments consisting of daily oral medication as well as injections once weekly. These treatments would continue for one full year.

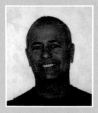

Tony Rahar

The problem is that the treatments while ongoing do not allow people to function normally. Being a husband, a father of a son who plays college football, and the sole provider for our family, I was reluctant to start the treatments

After long walks with my wife and extensive prayer, I was looking for an alternate plan to fight this disease. A friend and business associate suggested I seek the services of Chris Johnson. I have known Chris for many years and occasionally have sought out his services as a personal trainer. I have heard Chris's information before, but this time I was ready to listen! After meeting with Chris for over two hours I came away with a plan of action.

Starting with healthy foods, portion size, meal timing, a balance of healthy fats, carbohydrates, proteins, and a few supplements, my mind and body started to change. Within four months I lost twenty-eight pounds! I have a substantial increase in energy, a stronger resilience to stress, and an overall positive outlook regarding my health. But the best part is that my latest blood tests show my liver enzymes have changed from a dangerous level to normal. My doctors are enthused and have encouraged me to continue following Chris's program.

Chris Johnson's plan has changed my life. These changes are now my daily habits and will be forever. My family and I are eternally grateful to Chris for all of his guidance and compassion.

Chapter 4
HEALTHY CELLS ARE HAPPY CELLS

For years we have been influenced to focus on *calories* as the most important factor of food. Most people believe that to lose weight they just need to eat fewer calories. This may be true when starting a diet, but over time calorie restriction can lead to a feeling of deprivation, making the diet difficult to sustain. Imagine shifting your mindset away from calories and focusing on feeding your cells with *higher-quality food* that retains all its nutrients! For many, this can be difficult at first. The question I hear over and over is, "How many calories should I be eating per day? Is it 1,200 calories, 1,800 calories, 2,500 calories, or more?" My response: "It depends." It depends on many factors, but most of all it depends on the *quality* of the calories you are consuming.

> We don't know who we are until we see what we can do.
>
> —Martha Grimes

Once people "get" this concept, the way they look at food changes forever. No longer are they concerned about adding an extra 100 to 200 calories per day of healthy fat to their diets. Their attention has shifted away from calories and losing weight to feeding their cells high-quality foods and getting healthier. Their skin begins to look better, energy improves, clothes fit differently, cholesterol improves, blood glucose improves, their cells are slowly transforming, and the body is getting healthier!

One comment I hear on a regular basis from many of my personal training clients is how their skin is softer, their nails are growing faster, and their hair and scalp are much healthier due to eating higher-quality foods and beverages. Consuming higher-quality foods and beverages creates healthier and happier cells!

What about taste? "Do I need to eat wheat grass, cod liver oil, or sea vegetables to keep my cells in good shape?" You may want to do this in the future, but for now you don't need to worry about it. Whew! Okay, back to the cell. Our focus now turns to how we get healthy cells that result in healthy bodies.

The human body has over 100 trillion cells. One of the most beautiful aspects of the human body is its ability to adapt and heal itself. Each day the cells in the human body are going through constant change. In fact, *the human body turns over three to four trillion cells per day.* Each and every day you have a wonderful opportunity to improve your cellular health!

Most people have been taught that if you eat less and exercise more, weight loss is sure to follow. But there is more to it than just eating fewer calories and exercising more. Bonnie Klinger realized this firsthand. Bonnie was tired, overweight, and unhealthy. She thought she was doing all the right things to lose weight, but her plan was not working. When she finally understood that she needed to get her cells healthy first, everything else started to click. Her skin improved, she had more energy, her health improved, and she started losing weight. She had shifted her focus from how many calories she was eating to improving the quality of the food and beverages she was consuming. You don't need a college degree in chemistry or physiology to understand the cell, just learn a few basic principles. Getting healthy at the cellular level can change your life. It did for Bonnie.

THE CELL MEMBRANE

Let's begin with a better understanding of the cell. Every cell has an outer crust called the cell membrane. The main job of the cell membrane is to control what goes in and out of the cell. Keeping the cell membrane soft and permeable is critical to the overall health of every cell. *The goal is to get your cell membranes soft and permeable, and keep them soft and permeable as you age.*

Consuming high-quality foods and beverages, especially the right types of fats, is essential for keeping the cell membranes soft and healthy. If you consume processed foods and foods that contain trans-fats (partially hydrogenated oils), cell membranes start to become hard and brittle. Remember the M&M candy, hard on the outside and soft on the inside? That's how your cells may become if you don't take care of them. Hard and brittle cell membranes make it difficult for nutrients to enter the cells and for the cells to be fed correctly.

When we eat, blood glucose begins to rise and the hormone insulin is secreted to allow the cells to be fed. It

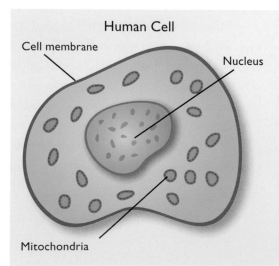

Human Cell

Cell membrane

Nucleus

Mitochondria

is insulin's job to open the cells for feeding. If a cell is hard and brittle, insulin has a hard time doing its job. Over time, the cell may become desensitized to insulin, leading to elevated blood glucose and even Type 2 diabetes.

One of the fastest-growing medical concerns we face in the United States is Type 2 diabetes. The major reason Type 2 diabetes is growing so quickly is directly related to the quality and quantity of the foods and beverages we consume. The major villain in the Type 2 diabetes epidemic is our overconsumption of trans-fats. Trans-fats make cell membranes hard and brittle, making it extremely difficult for insulin to penetrate them. *Your first step in getting your cells soft and healthy is to get the trans-fats out of your diet and begin to replace them with healthy fats.* Healthy fats make the cell membrane soft and receptive to insulin. Regular exercise also improves the health and receptiveness of the cell membrane. Over time you don't need to produce as much insulin because the cell is more receptive so the need for Type 2 diabetes medications may slowly begin to disappear. I will go into more detail about fats in Chapter 12.

MITOCHONDRIA

Another essential part of the cell is the mitochondria. The mitochondria are the power pack of the cell, equivalent to the engine of a car. The performance of the mitochondria in the cell is directly related to how your body uses energy. The more active the mitochondria, the more calories your body will use for energy. In each cell there are hundreds to thousands of mitochondria. The number and activity level of each mitochondrion are directly related to a healthy lifestyle! Genetics does play a role, but it is small in comparison to healthy lifestyle practices.

Many of the clients I see tell me that they have a stubborn metabolism. They are exercising more than ever and eating well, but can't seem to lose weight. When we discuss their food log, I usually see a diet that is low in calories, but missing the essential fats needed to fuel the mitochondria. I tell them they need to feed the mitochondria correctly so the cells can become more active.

The first step in getting the mitochondria healthy is to drink more water, eat more fruits and vegetables, and most of all, feed the mitochondria the right types of fat. This is another of the many reasons why consuming the right types of fats is essential for optimal health and weight control.

NUCLEUS OF THE CELL

Last but not least is the nucleus of the cell. The nucleus is the core and brain center of the cell. It orchestrates communication throughout the entire human body. Each cell also has a genetic makeup that determines everything from the color of our eyes and hair to the length of our bones. We can do little to change our genetic makeup, but that doesn't play as big a role in the outcome of our health and how we feel as we once thought.

You can make a huge impact on your health and how you feel every day by improving the quality of the food you eat and what you drink. Can you imagine trying to build a house with poor-quality raw materials? The same can be said of the human body. If you don't feed your cells the right raw materials, how can you produce a healthy outcome within the body?

Change your mindset away from how many calories you are consuming. Focus on improving the *quality* of your food and drink choices. *Focus on getting healthier at the cellular level!* As your cells become healthier, you will begin to have better health and more energy, improved sleep, less inflammation, and that stubborn waistline that wasn't getting any smaller will begin to magically shrink.

THE BOTTOM LINE

1. The human body has over 100 trillion cells and 3–4 trillion of these cells turn over each day!
2. The cell membrane is the outer crust of the cell and acts as the gatekeeper of the cell, controlling what goes in and out of the cell.
3. The mitochondria are the power pack of the cell and play a large role in how your body uses energy.
4. The nucleus is the center of the cell and orchestrates communication throughout the entire human body.
5. What we choose to eat and drink is a major factor in determining the health of our cells.

Chapter 5
ALKALINE/ACID:
BALANCING THE BODY'S pH

Do you remember the old Alka-Seltzer™ commercial, "Plop, Plop, Fizz, Fizz, Oh What a Relief It Is"? If you had heartburn (acid reflux) or stomach discomfort, Alka-Seltzer™ was the over-the-counter medication of choice to relieve your discomfort.

Nothing liberates our greatness like the desire to serve.

—Marianne Williamson

This commercial was extremely popular around the holiday season when we have a tendency to overindulge. What magical ingredient in Alka-Seltzer™ helped decrease your heartburn or stomach discomfort? That ingredient is sodium bicarbonate. Sodium bicarbonate is extremely alkaline, hence the name Alka-Seltzer™.

Here comes a little chemistry lesson. Just stay focused on the concept, and it will make more sense as we go along. Interest in alkaline/acid balance and its role in maintaining optimal health has been growing. Alkalinity and acidity are measured in pH (potential of hydrogen).

Every food and beverage has an acid or alkaline characteristic and is measured on a pH scale of zero to fourteen, with zero being the most acidic and fourteen the most alkaline. For example, the pH of stomach acid is 1, diet soda pop is 2.5, coffee is 3, water is 7 (neutral), venous blood is 7.35, arterial blood is 7.45, sea water is 8.5, and baking soda is 12 (similar to Alka-Seltzer™). You can monitor your pH on a regular basis by the use of litmus strips. These may be purchased at most health food stores or pharmacies and measure the pH of your saliva or urine. *Ideally, the human blood pH should be slightly alkaline, between 7.35 and 7.45.* The pH of your saliva and urine should fall between 6.8 and 7.2.

Foods and beverages are classified as acid-forming or alkalizing depending on the effect they have on the body. An *acid-forming* food or beverage *adds hydrogen* ions to the body, making it more acidic. An *alkalizing* food or beverage *removes hydrogen* ions from the body, making it more alkaline. *The classification of whether a food or beverage is acid or alkaline is based on the effect it has on the body after digestion or the end-product of digestion.* For example, lemons are extremely acidic; however, the end-products they produce after digestion are more alkaline, making lemons alkaline-forming in the body. A simple way to increase the alkalinity of a glass of water is to add a slice of lemon or lime.

One last item before this all comes together: just because a food or beverage is acid-forming does not mean it is unhealthy! Blueberries and walnuts are examples of acid-forming foods, but they also have many wonderful health benefits.

Your body won't allow your pH to become unbalanced. If it did, you would die. But when your body has to work overtime to maintain a balanced pH, the trouble begins! This is primarily due to the overconsumption of acid-forming foods and beverages and unhealthy stress. We consume considerably more acid-forming than alkaline-forming foods and beverages. We consume too much coffee, caffeine, soda pop, beer, alcohol, processed foods, fried foods, high-fructose corn syrup, sugar, artificial sweeteners, and animal proteins, just to name a few. On top of our unhealthy food and beverage choices, we live in a world that keeps speeding up, which may lead to high levels of unhealthy stress.

Health problems related to an acid-forming diet and high levels of stress	
acid reflux	osteoporosis
irritable bowel syndrome	inflammation
stomach discomfort	dry skin
insomnia	cracked nails
headaches	premature aging
fatigue	cardiovascular damage
muscle cramps	diabetes
constipation	thyroid dysfunction
kidney stones	weight gain

HOW DO AN ACID-FORMING DIET AND HIGH LEVELS OF STRESS LEAD TO ALL OF THESE HEALTH PROBLEMS?

One thing I find fascinating about the human body is its ability to fix itself through endless checks and balances. This is especially evident with blood pH. If the pH of the blood starts to become unbalanced in either direction by the smallest of margins, the body quickly brings it back into balance through a number of buffering systems. These buffering systems include the lungs, blood, kidneys, and minerals. As the blood becomes too acidic (less than 7.3), mechanisms kick in to bring blood pH back to 7.4. The rate of breathing will increase to remove carbonic acid by exhaling carbon dioxide, the kidneys increase the acidity of the urine, minerals begin to be leached out of the body, and, quickly, blood pH is back to normal.

To compensate for an acid-forming diet and high levels of stress, the body uses alkaline-forming minerals such as calcium, magnesium, iodine, potassium, and sodium. As the pH in the body becomes more acidic, these alkaline-forming minerals are used to buffer the high acid level. These minerals work in the blood, lymphatic system, and extracellular and intracellular fluids to bind acids, which are then removed through the urine. Over time these minerals may become depleted, leading to myriad health problems.

It sounds like the body has all the checks and balances in place to maintain a balanced blood pH, so what's the big deal? If we abuse our bodies with poor food and beverage choices, with little or no exercise and high levels of unhealthy stress, *the body can only do so much over time before the effort starts to take its toll!*

One of the fastest-growing groups of medications in the United States is medications that relieve acid reflux. These medications may help to relieve the discomfort, but are they truly fixing the problem? You may want to ask yourself, "Why do I have acid reflux to begin with?" I have witnessed many who have completely done away with their acid reflux medications by improving the quality of the foods and beverages they consume. Remember how Alka-Seltzer™ helped to relieve acid reflux? By including more alkaline-forming foods and beverages in your diet you give your body what it needs to heal itself, and your acid reflux slowly disappears!

Other health problems may also be linked to an acid-forming diet. In the United States we have one of the highest intakes of calcium in the world, but still have poor bone health when compared with other countries. Doesn't that statement make you stand up and ask why? If we are consuming enough calcium to keep our bones healthy, what seems to be the problem? One of the real culprits in the United States is our overconsumption of beverages that are acid-forming in the body, such as soda pop, coffee, energy drinks, and alcohol.

To give you an idea of how powerful some of these beverages can be, let's do a simple experiment. You have a little rust on the bumper of your classic car, so you take a rag, pour some soda pop on the rag, add a little elbow grease, and off comes the rust! The ingredient in soda pop that takes off the rust is phosphoric acid. Drinking too much soda pop creates an acid environment in the body. As the pH slowly begins to shift to the acid side, the body goes to work calling on its buffering systems to bring the pH back to normal. Minerals such as calcium play a large role in the buffering process, so over time calcium may be leached from the body, causing weak bones. If the soda pop can take the rust off a car bumper, imagine how some of these acid-forming beverages can affect your bone health over time!

Another area of concern in the United States is thyroid problems, especially among women. Over 20 percent of all women over the age of fifty in the United States have reported thyroid problems! Many women over the age of fifty report feeling tired, with dry skin, intolerance to cold, muscle aches, depression, and an increase in body fat.

What does pH have to do with thyroid problems? One of the main functions of the thyroid gland is to control metabolism. If you have an under-producing thyroid gland, your metabolism can become sluggish and weight gain may follow. The mineral iodine helps to support the thyroid gland. Your iodine reserves, just like your calcium reserves, may become depleted over time if your pH is out of balance due to unhealthy stress, lack of rest, lack of exercise, and poor food and beverage choices. Remember, your thyroid gland plays a large role in your metabolism. This is one reason why diet soft drinks that contain zero calories may indirectly cause a person to gain weight. How can a diet soft drink that contains no calories cause weight gain? I missed that. Most soda pop contains phosphoric acid, which increases the acid in the body. Over time, valuable minerals are slowly leached out of the body, including the mineral iodine, and iodine helps support the thyroid gland. So, if your body depletes your mineral reserves, your thyroid gland, along with the overall health of the entire body, begins to suffer.

Foods high in iodine include:	
agar	kale
artichokes	leafy greens
asparagus	oats
blueberries	onions
brussels sprouts	sea vegetables
carrots	squash
coconut	strawberries
cucumbers	sweet potatoes
eggplant	tofu
fish	tomatoes
goat's milk	watermelon
green peppers	

I find it interesting that women in Japan have wonderful bone health and virtually no thyroid problems, yet only consume 300–400 mg of calcium per day. Their diet is made up of highly alkaline foods such as fish, leafy greens, tofu, and sea vegetables. Sea vegetables! What are sea vegetables? Sushi nori, arame, and dulse are different types of sea vegetables that are extremely high in iodine. (My favorite is sushi nori. I use it to wrap sandwiches or crumble it on a salad.) Sea water is highly alkaline, so it makes sense that vegetables grown in the sea are highly alkaline and also high in iodine. Now wait a minute, I'm not saying you have to eat sea vegetables! Sea vegetables can wait for now, but eating more fruits, vegetables, and healthy fats, and drinking more water and controlling stress can help move your body's pH to the alkaline side.

WHAT CAUSES ACID AND ALKALINE TO BECOME UNBALANCED?

High levels of stress and negative emotions

Nothing moves the body to become acidic faster than excessive stress and negative emotions. Excessive stress and negative emotions can mean many things to many people. When your life begins to get out of balance (working too much, bills to pay, lack of sleep, little or no exercise, eating unhealthy foods, problems at home or work), getting your life back into balance can be challenging. In our 24/7 world we all get out of balance now and then; at least I do. The challenge is how to get yourself back in balance and improve your thinking. Do you perceive your circumstances from a positive or negative standpoint? In the book *Power vs. Force*, David R. Hawkins, M.D., Ph.D., describes how your perceptions, attitudes, and even your word associations affect your energy fields. Thoughts of peace, joy, and acceptance have much higher energy fields than thoughts of anger, guilt, or shame, which have low energy fields. This is not meant to be a section on psychology or stress management; my point is for you to understand how excessive stress and negative emotions can trigger the hormones adrenaline and cortisol. Adrenaline and cortisol accelerate acid levels throughout the body, which may lead to mineral loss.

Eating too much protein

Proteins are acidic in nature. Consuming more than 25 percent of your daily calories from protein may cause the body to become acidic. Also, consuming non-organic animal sources of proteins may increase the acidity level in the body due to high levels of antibiotics fed to animals. Twenty years ago we didn't have to worry about consuming non-organic animal sources of proteins, but now it is a much greater concern. Many animals are raised to grow faster and larger by being fed growth hormones. As the animals begin to grow at abnormally fast rates, the risk of contracting diseases increases. To shut down disease in these animals, the animals are also fed antibiotics.

Consuming foods that contain antibiotics and hormones is not good for the human body. First, consuming foods that contain hormones and antibiotics may upset the natural balance of bacteria in the stomach. Antibiotics can damage the naturally occurring bacteria in the stomach that are essential for proper digestion and absorption of nutrients, which may then lead to digestive problems such as acid reflux and irritable bowel syndrome. Second, antibiotics are highly acidic. So, by consuming too much protein, especially from non-organic animal sources, the body becomes even more acidic. This can result in critical minerals becoming depleted.

High dietary intake of phosphates/phosphoric acid

Foods such as processed cheeses, ice cream, artificial sweeteners, fried foods, beef, cocoa, sugar, table salt, and cottage cheese create high acid levels. Beverages such as colas, coffee, and beer also increase acid levels.

WHAT CAN I DO TO BALANCE MY ACID AND ALKALINE LEVELS?

Consume foods that have high alkaline levels

Most fruits and vegetables have high alkaline levels and help maintain alkaline-acid balance. Sea vegetables are one of the best sources of iodine and are extremely alkaline. Oatmeal is one of the highest-alkaline whole grains. Most healthy fats such as extra-virgin olive oil, cod liver oil, almonds, and flaxseeds are highly alkaline.

I am often asked in my seminars whether salt is good or bad. The answer is, *"it depends!"* It depends on the *quality* of the salt. Are you asking about sea salt, which is highly alkaline, or are you asking about table salt, which is highly acidic? Is there really that big a difference between the types of salt you are consuming? Absolutely! So if you like using salt, sea salt is a much better choice. This is another example of how to make simple choices that improve the quality of your food.

Consume beverages that have high alkaline levels

Coffee is usually acidic. However, consuming higher-quality coffee, such as an organic coffee, or moving to a healthier beverage choice, such as green tea, can improve the pH. Drinking mineral water and adding a slice of lemon to your water are excellent ways to help balance your pH. Non-dairy milk choices such as almond milk are alkaline options versus the more acidic cow's milk. Start slowly to improve the quality of your drink sources.

Rest and recovery

Take time for yourself. Get more sleep. Take regular vacations. Try to get a little down time each day. Change your breathing patterns. Taking deep, slow breaths for thirty to sixty seconds, spread out a few times over your day, can help to reduce stress. These will all improve your health and the pH balance in your body.

pH table						
	Most alkaline	**More alkaline**	**Least alkaline**	**Least acidic**	**More acidic**	**Most acidic**
Condiments, spices, sweeteners	baking soda, sea salt	cinnamon, most spices, molasses	most herbs, rice syrup	curry, honey, maple syrup, stevia/agave nectar	vanilla, MSG, Splenda, organic sugar	nutmeg, table salt, pudding, jam, jelly, artificial sweeteners, sugar, cocoa
Beverages	mineral water, lemon/lime water	spring/artesian water, green tea	tap water, ginger tea	purified water, white tea, organic coffee, red wine	distilled water, black tea, white wine	soda pop, energy drinks, coffee, alcohol/beer
Dairy		human breast milk, almond milk	ghee, rice/oat milk	butter, yogurt, soy/goat milk, goat cheese	casein, organic cow's milk, cottage cheese	ice cream, cow's milk, processed cheese
Meat/seafood/eggs			fish	shrimp, turkey/chicken, game meat, eggs	pork/veal, lean red meat	lobster, hot dogs, deli meat, fast-food burgers
Grains/cereal			wild rice, quinoa, oats	brown rice, amaranth, millet, kashi	wheat, white rice, rye, spelt	barley, corn
Nuts/oils	pumpkin seeds	almonds, cod liver oil, evening primrose oil, sesame seeds	flaxseed oil, extra-virgin olive oil, organic coconut oil, most seeds	pine nuts, safflower oil, almond/canola oil	sesame oil, peanuts	pecans, brazil nuts, palm kernel oil, fried food, lard, walnuts
Beans/legumes	lentils			pinto beans, lima beans, kidney beans	navy/red beans, white beans, split peas, beans, most legumes	soybeans, tempeh, chickpeas
Vegetables	sea vegetables, broccoli, yams barley grass, wheat grass, asparagus, sweet potato, kale, parsley	eggplant, bell peppers, cauliflower, collard greens, cabbage, garlic, sprouts, pumpkin	squash, lettuce, beets, brussels sprouts, cucumber, celery, potato	spinach, zucchini, string beans	peas, carrots	
Fruits	lime, pineapple, nectarine, watermelon, raspberries, tangerine	apple, kiwi, peach, blackberries, grapefruit, melon, mango, lemon, avocado	orange, banana, blueberries, raisins, grapes, strawberries	dry fruit, figs, dates, plum, coconut	prune, tomatoes, pomegranate, cranberries	
Lifestyle	sleep, deep breathing, massage, joy, love, enlightenment, bliss, peace	optimism, forgiveness, balanced exercise, hope, kindness	willingness, courage, pride	pomposity, confusion, forcefulness, demeaning	sedentary lifestyle, lack of sleep, unhealthy stress, overwork	guilt, shame, fear, blame, apathy

To maintain a balanced pH, shoot for 65 to 70 percent of all your food and beverage sources coming from the alkaline portion of the pH table.

THE BOTTOM LINE

1. Alkaline/acid is measured by relative pH in blood. Your pH can be easily measured by using a litmus strip to test your urine or saliva.
2. Lack of exercise, too much stress, and a highly acidic diet may lead to excessive stress on the body's buffering systems.
3. The body balances pH through many buffering systems including the lungs, blood, kidneys, and alkaline minerals.
4. Many health problems in the United States can be linked to an acid-forming diet and high levels of stress.
5. Try to consume 65 to 70 percent of your foods and beverages from alkaline sources and control unhealthy stress to keep an acid/alkaline balance.

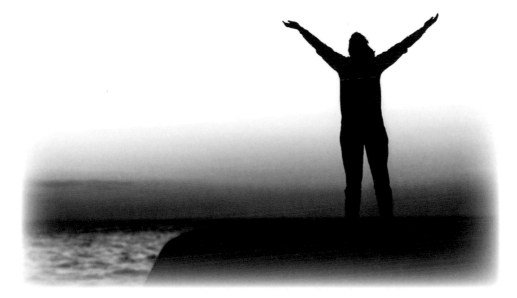

TAKE IT FROM ME...

Here is my story. I have a heart valve disorder. Seven years ago at the age of thirty-six, I was suffering from symptoms of this disorder that caused me to be in bed each day exhausted by 4:00 p.m., among other various discomforts. The fatigue was the worst, as I felt I was losing so much time with my kids and husband. I weighed 170 pounds at the time and I am five feet two inches tall, so obviously the weight was a big part in worsening my symptoms. My cardiologist wanted me to start walking to increase my activity level. I never realized that I was getting heavy. I was raising young kids and felt I had been active. I also felt I ate "pretty well." I was not even close to either, I later realized. I began to walk as recommended. Then after several months and a bit of progress, I started taking group fitness classes. I continued to slowly lose weight. I added some kickboxing, then strength training. I loved it! I was hooked on exercise and it became a lifestyle change. I even became certified to teach group fitness, to help others become passionate about exercise.

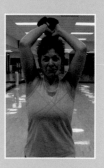

Tina Brookhouse, Group Fitness Instructor

During this time I was taking a heart medication to help the blood flow through the heart with less stress to the heart. The doctor said I would be on this medication for life, as the valve disorder was not reversible, and would progress as I aged. At some point a valve replacement would more than likely be in store for me. The doctor was, however, pleased with my progress of losing thirty pounds in the first three years of my exercise regimen. Still, the weight was slow to come off and my weight loss had plateaued for over a year. My total cholesterol was 247 and my HDL and LDL cholesterol were also not too good.

Then I was introduced to On Target Living when I became employed as a group fitness instructor at the Michigan Athletic Club. I started taking healthy fats. I took all the corn syrup and hydrogenated oils out of my diet. I also deleted all the white, refined sugar and flour. I ate every three hours. My energy skyrocketed. I added high-intensity training to my exercise regimen as well as group cycling, core classes, and running 5K races! In nine months I lost twenty pounds. On Target Living was the catalyst I had been missing. Combining the exercise with the new way of eating was the key. What had taken years to lose, came off so much faster. The science behind Chris Johnson's book really works. My good cholesterol came up twenty points, my bad cholesterol came down forty-seven points. My weight went from 170 pounds to 128 pounds. But my favorite part is: in my last cardiologist visit, my doctor took me off the medication that he was sure I would be on forever!! My doctor was amazed, and said I am a poster child for what he wishes all of his patients would do. Thanks, Chris!

Chapter 6
GOING ORGANIC

What's all the fuss about organic foods? Is there a benefit to eating more organic foods? As more people become educated on the importance of quality food, the demand for organic food will continue to rise.

Organic foods and beverages are the fastest-growing segment of the U.S. food market, growing at more than 20 percent per year and projected to reach more than $35 billion in sales by 2008. In 1990, the U.S. Congress passed the Organic Food Production Act, which ordered the U.S. Department of Agriculture to set certification standards for the production, processing, and certification of organic food. In 2002, these criteria were finalized by the Organic Foods Standards Act.

> **Life is an adventure in forgiveness.**
>
> —Norman Cousins

WHAT DOES "ORGANIC" MEAN?

Organic food is produced without using pesticides, antibiotics, and fertilizers made from synthetic ingredients. Organic meat, poultry, eggs, and dairy products come from animals that are not fed or given pesticides, fertilizers, steroids, growth hormones, or antibiotics.

HOW DO YOU KNOW IT'S ORGANIC?

This is an area in which the government has helped. In 2002, the USDA officially divided organic products into four categories requiring producers and manufacturers to correctly label their products.

- **100-percent organic:** Product states that all of its ingredients are completely organic.
- **Organic:** Product states that at least 95 percent of its contents are organic by weight.
- **Made with organic ingredients:** Product states that at least 70 percent of its contents are organic.
- **Less than 70 percent of the content is organic:** Product may list only those ingredients that are organic on the ingredient panel.

HOW MUCH DOES IT COST?

Buying organic foods and beverages does cost more, on average between 10 and 30 percent more. One of the main reasons that organic foods are more expensive is that they are not subsidized, so consumers are paying more for the cost of growing, processing, and shipping, and also preserving the integrity of our land and water sources.

You don't have to move to eating all organic foods overnight. I recommend moving to more *organic animal products first,* due to the growth hormones and antibiotics given to our conventionally raised animals. Choosing organic eggs and dairy is a great place to start. You can now buy organic eggs and dairy products in most conventional grocery stores. Organic meat sources may be a bit more challenging to find, but there is a large movement to provide more meat products at lower prices. Buying more organic fruits, vegetables, and whole grains is important, due to the pesticides and synthetic fertilizers used, but choosing organic animal products is the best place to start in your organic food journey!

As the demand for higher-quality food sources continues to climb, more and more stores will offer a variety of organic foods and beverages. Start slowly and enjoy the difference organic foods can make.

TAKE IT FROM ME...

I was not satisfied with the way that I looked. I had been working out regularly and eating a fairly healthy diet but felt stuck at a certain level. After attending one of Chris's On Target Living seminars, I decided that I wanted to go to the next level of fitness and health at the age of sixty. How far I could go I did not know, so I hired the services of Chris Johnson to guide me. Today at the age of sixty-three, I have gone to the next level of nutrition, while enjoying food in a new and exciting way, and I have learned to enjoy my workouts with greater precision, exactness, and enthusiasm, and I have remained injury free. I am extremely happy with the results. I have lost over twenty pounds and have maintained my current weight of 172 pounds with a body fat of 14 percent for over two years. I look forward to the next level, whatever that might be.

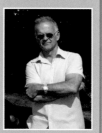

Gary Wood

THE BOTTOM LINE

1. Organic foods and beverages are the fastest-growing segment of the U.S. food market, growing at more than 20 percent per year.
2. Organic food is produced without using pesticides, antibiotics, and fertilizers made from synthetic products.
3. In 2002, the USDA officially divided organic products into four categories: 100-percent organic, organic, made with organic ingredients, less than 70 percent of the content is organic.
4. Buying organic foods and beverages costs an average of 10 to 30 percent more.
5. Start slowly and enjoy the difference organic foods can make.

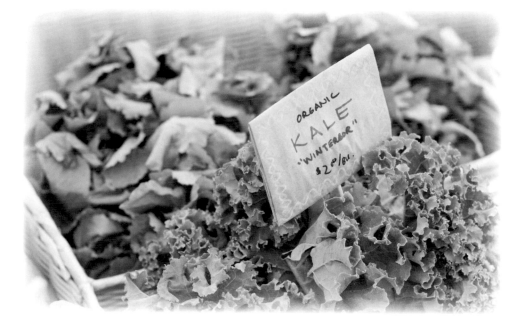

Chapter 7
LAYING THE FOUNDATION

We all want to feel good and have good health! As the saying goes, "when you don't have your health you don't have anything," and this is so true. What do good health and performance look like? It could be as simple as having more energy throughout your day, getting up in the morning with fewer aches and pains, decreasing the amount of medications that you are currently taking, climbing a flight of stairs with less effort, having greater mental focus at work or at school, performing better on the athletic field, having more pep in your step, or just plain feeling your best!

> The ripest peach is highest on the tree.
>
> —James Whitcomb Riley

Most people want to feel good and perform their best in whatever they do. Wouldn't you like to have this feeling on a more consistent basis? You can create a consistent pattern of feeling your best every day!

MASLOW'S HIERARCHY OF HUMAN NEEDS

A few years ago, I became fascinated with Abraham Maslow's Hierarchy of Human Needs. Maslow, a psychologist, created his hierarchy based on what he learned from his studies with monkeys. Maslow discovered that certain needs take precedence over others. The monkeys would not move up the hierarchy of needs until the needs of the preceding level were met. For example, if the monkeys were thirsty, drinking water would take precedence over eating, and up the hierarchy they would go. Maslow then laid out five levels of human needs—Physiological Needs, Safety Needs, Belonging Needs, Esteem Needs and Self-Actualization Needs.

Maslow calls the first four levels of needs deficit needs, meaning if you don't have

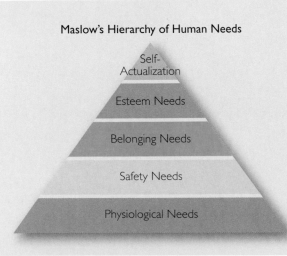

Maslow's Hierarchy of Human Needs

Self-Actualization

Esteem Needs

Belonging Needs

Safety Needs

Physiological Needs

enough of something you have a deficit, so you feel a need. The highest level of Maslow's Hierarchy of Human Needs is Self-Actualization. This level is where the fun begins. These are needs that do not involve balance. The more attention we give these needs, the stronger they become. They involve the continuous desire to fulfill potentials, to "be all you can be." The catch is that if you truly want to be self-actualizing, you need to take care of your deficit needs first.

You might be thinking, "What does Maslow's Hierarchy of Human Needs have to do with a book on nutrition?" I am always fascinated when I listen to people express their needs—working on a new career, making more money, developing personal relationships, buying a new house…the list goes on and on. In our hurried society some of the most basic physiological human needs are often neglected. For many, taking care of these fundamental needs is not even on the radar screen. We seem to have forgotten that it is difficult to perform at our best when we don't get enough sleep, eat poorly, and rarely move our bodies.

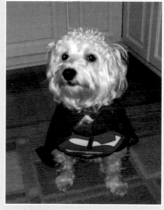

The most consistent creature at following the hierarchy of needs is my dog, Dolly. Dolly has the dog hierarchy of needs down to a science! Granted, Dolly does not have a job or many responsibilities, but she does have her rituals in place to take care of her hierarchy of needs. The first thing Dolly does when she gets up in the morning is her up-and-down dog stretch, followed by a strong desire to go outside and do her business. She then comes into the house and gets a drink of water, followed by eating her food. She then moves up her hierarchy of needs and wants to play.

Building a stronger foundation can be easier than you think. Start slowly, make small changes, and "be all you can be"!

THE THREE BUILDING BLOCKS OF YOUR FOUNDATION

The three basic ingredients that form the foundation of Maslow's Hierarchy of Human Needs are **Rest and Recovery, Nutrition,** and **Movement or Exercise.** You can't build a strong house unless you have a solid foundation; the same is true for the human body. A few basic principles can keep our bodies healthy and performing at the top of our game. Be kind to yourself, take care of the basics, and enjoy life!

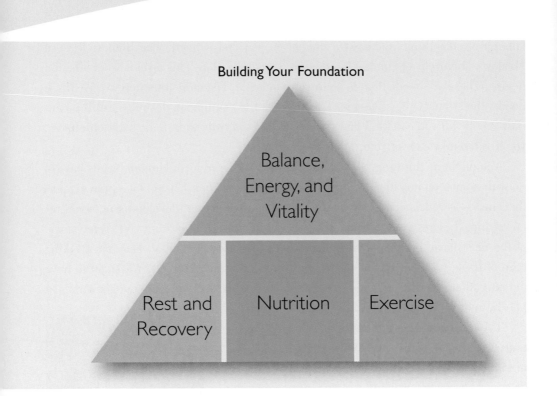

Building Your Foundation

Balance, Energy, and Vitality

Rest and Recovery | Nutrition | Exercise

I. Rest/recovery

When consulting with individual clients or speaking to large audiences through my seminars, I like to begin with rest/recovery as the foundation for feeling your best. Getting enough rest is critical for good health and performing at your best. Have you ever taken a vacation and within just a few days found that your quality of sleep started to improve, your energy was better, and you started feeling like your old self again? We are a sleep-deprived nation, with a high percentage of our population getting less than six hours of sleep per night on a regular basis.

Many countries around the world have rest and recovery plugged into their normal daily routine. Many countries actually shut down for a few hours every afternoon. It gives them time to eat and rest. In the United States everything is on 24/7. We all need more down time to rest and recharge our batteries!

Without enough rest the adrenal gland becomes overstimulated, secreting too much of the stress hormone cortisol. High levels of cortisol can break down the body in many ways, leading to problems such as weight gain, low energy, high blood pressure, depression, inflammation, osteoporosis, low thyroid, heart attacks, and decreased immune function, to name a few.

Many people come to see me because they want to lose weight. When I begin talking about their sleep patterns or what type of recovery habits they use, they get this quizzical look on their face. "Why are you talking about sleep? I am here to learn how to exercise and lose weight."

I explain to them that proper rest, especially their quality of sleep, is directly related to weight loss and better health. Your digestive system has two hormones that control hunger and appetite: *ghrelin* and *leptin*. Ghrelin is secreted by the stomach and sends out a signal that you are hungry. Lack of sleep stimulates the hormone ghrelin, which plays a role in making you want to overeat. Leptin plays the opposite role to that of ghrelin. Leptin tells the brain that you are satisfied. If you are getting enough restful sleep your body will secrete leptin, letting your brain know that you are satisfied, having less desire to overeat.

Ideally, the human body needs *between seven and eight hours of sleep each night.* The challenge becomes how to get the rest needed to feel your best. Here are a few rest and recovery patterns to start with.

Set up a ritual in which you plan your sleep patterns

Go to bed at the same time each night and get up at the same time each morning. Give yourself the time necessary to get a full night's rest. When changing time zones it takes the body a few days to begin to acclimate to new sleep patterns. The same can be true for developing healthier sleep patterns at home. Planning bedtime is a great place to start. If you have to get up each day at 5:30 a.m., then try to be in bed no later than 10:30 p.m. each night. Setting up consistent bedtime patterns will allow the body and mind to function at their best.

Create a restful environment

Start by making sure your bedroom is completely dark. Even the lights from an illuminated clock create light. If you have trouble with noise distractions try using white noise, such as a small fan, a bedside waterfall, or a noise machine to create the restful environment you need. If you have trouble falling or staying asleep, avoid watching television for an hour before going to bed. Instead, read a book to let the brain slow down. I tell my clients they may want to pick up my book and read a chapter if they are having trouble falling asleep—it works every time!

Pay attention to what you eat or drink before bedtime

Avoid eating a big meal at least one to two hours before going to bed. Also, avoid alcohol, caffeine, and if possible any medications that may interfere with sleep.

Change your breathing patterns

One of the fastest ways to help slow down and get rest and recovery during the day is to change your breathing patterns. When people are upset, stressed, or nervous, they change the way they breathe. Watch a basketball player at the free throw line with one second on the clock remaining and down by a point. Observe how they try to change the way they breathe to help them relax. They take slow deep breaths. By taking slow, deep breaths, the phrenic nerve above the diaphragm is stimulated, signaling the brain to slow down, followed by a drop in blood pressure and heart rate.

Next time you feel stressed or need a little time to recover, take a few slow, deep breaths. You may even want to build a few breathing breaks into your day. Find a quiet place with no interruptions, close your eyes, and take slow deep breaths. I advise many of my personal training clients to plug in sixty-second deep-breathing breaks to help control their stress and give them a chance to recover throughout their day. It is amazing how sixty seconds of slow, deep breathing can make you feel.

Don't underestimate the power that adequate rest and recovery can give you!

2. Nutrition

The second building block of your foundation for better health and performance is high-quality nutrition. As a society we underestimate the impact that healthy nutrition has on the human body. The specifics of nutrition will be discussed in greater detail in Section 2.

3. Movement/exercise

The third building block of your foundation is movement/exercise. The human body is designed to move. If there was such a thing as "the fountain of youth," regular exercise would be at the top of the list. Moving your body is one of the fastest ways to change your mood. When presenting seminars to large audiences, I find ways to get everyone moving when I feel the need to change the energy in the room. Just by adding movement, such as standing and waving arms, laughter begins, smiles appear, and the energy of an entire room changes. *Motion creates positive emotion!*

The specifics of exercise will be discussed in greater detail in Chapter 26.

THE BOTTOM LINE

1. Abraham Maslow's Hierarchy of Human Needs: Physiological, Safety, Belonging, Esteem, Self-Actualization
2. Getting enough sleep (seven to eight hours per night), along with short bouts of recovery during your day, is critical for optimal health and performance.
3. Changing your breathing patterns (slow, deep breathing) is an easy and effective way to get more rest and recovery into your day.
4. What you feed your body is directly related to how you feel and perform.
5. Regular exercise is good for the body and mind. Motion creates positive emotion!

TAKE IT FROM ME...

The most challenging thing that I experience as a chiropractor dealing with patients is getting them to follow through with lifestyle changes. In my busy office, I unfortunately don't have the time necessary to focus a great deal of attention on people's diets and establishing exercise programs with them. Therefore, I do the basics: advise them, encourage them, and give them informational handouts. Handouts that I knew 90 percent of the time were never read and the information was never applied in their lives. It creates a very huge frustration for me, and a very large gap in how I was helping my patients.

Then I was introduced to Chris Johnson and his On Target Living program, and I found the perfect tool to fit my needs for nutritional and exercise education. I started out by having patients record their food intake and compare it to the *Food Target*. This allowed them to visualize how poorly they were eating. Seeing it on paper was very powerful and it seemed to spark an interest in them to make a change. I then had them read Chris's book.

I was overwhelmed by the response. Patients got the concept of making small changes over time, and then making more small changes. They would come into the office excited and tell me the changes they had made and what they were going to change next. I encouraged and motivated, but they were the ones educating themselves and then applying it to their lives. The program empowered them to take responsibility for their own health. As a doctor, that is a dream come true!

I highly recommend On Target Living to my patients and to other physicians who are looking for a way to empower their patients to make long-term healthy lifestyle changes.

Thank you, Chris.

—Dr. Scott Kribs

TAKE IT FROM ME...

For most of my adult life, I have struggled with my weight. I was the typical yo-yo dieter. I would gain weight, get disgusted with myself, go on a diet, lose weight, stop dieting when I achieved my "goal" weight, and begin the whole process over again and again and again. During these many years of yo-yo dieting, I became very focused on the numbers on the scale. When the numbers became too high, I experienced days and weeks of food deprivation. While I was depriving myself I would look forward to the day I hit the "right" number on the scale so I could begin eating again. My life was one vicious cycle of eating, which equated to weight gain followed by brief periods of deprivation, which equated to temporary weight loss. I had many different sizes of clothes in my closet, a size to fit whatever place in the cycle I happened to be in at any particular time. While I projected to the world that I was a joy-filled person, inside I was very down and out. I woke up every day thinking about how fat I was, how unfit I was, how I would start tomorrow. I was truly a hostage shackled in my own skin.

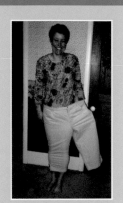

**Mary Heintzkill,
Borgess Medical Center,
Kalamazoo, Michigan**

Finally, in total desperation, I attended Chris Johnson's On Target Living Seminar in October 2004. At that point I was on the brink of disaster. I was nearing my fiftieth birthday. The years of yo-yo dieting were beginning to catch up with me. I weighed 236 pounds; my physician had recently put me on a blood pressure medication; my cholesterol was 230, and my triglycerides were quite elevated. Although I had begun walking three miles a day, I was still fat, unfit, and extremely unhealthy. When I attended Chris's seminar, I felt hope for the first time in years. One of Chris's main messages is to focus on making small changes. He made it clear that one change today and one change next week would eventually add up to big changes. He also wanted the audience to understand On Target Living was about making a choice for wellness. After his seminar, I realized that I needed to stop fighting my body and treat it like the gift that it was. This gift desperately wanted and needed to be nourished with a fuel worthy of a friend. I began to make the daily commitment to wellness, utilizing the principles set forth by Chris Johnson.

The journey that began with Chris's principles in October 2004 has had a tremendous impact on my life. Little by little, choice by choice, one step at a time, I began to add things to my overall health journey. I decided to try things that I never dreamed I would try. Actually, I dreamed of trying them, but was too embarrassed to try them. Who wants to see a really fat person in spandex shorts? Today, I exercise every day and I mix up my exercise routine with yoga, swimming, spinning, walking/running, and weight training. Along with the exercise, I decided to eat in the green areas of the On Target Living *Food Target*. Since I began aiming for the center of the *Food Target*, I have lost over seventy pounds. But the downward movement of the scale was not my primary objective. Remember that I was a healthcare disaster waiting to happen. My newfound friend, my body, began to respond positively to the gradual changes I was making. My blood pressure is now 90/60 without medication. My resting pulse is around 50, my cholesterol is 143, and my triglycerides are now in the healthy range.

Best of all, I have no intention of EVER, EVER dieting again. I am done with that. I need to thank Chris for encouraging me to get off the vicious cycle of yo-yo dieting. The shackles that once held me hostage have been removed. I am free. Thank you, Chris, for helping me liberate my body, mind, and spirit!

Chapter 8
LET FOOD
BE YOUR MEDICINE

In my more than two decades in the health and fitness industry, with over 15,000 hours of one-on-one personal training and speaking across the country in my On Target Living Seminars, an alarming message has come through—the United States has become an overmedicated society! Why are so many people looking for medications as the means to improve their health? Is it because we have more medications available? Are our doctors prescribing more medications? Do we have stronger advertising by the phar-

> Why treat an illness from a medicine bag versus curing it with food?
>
> —Hippocrates

maceutical companies? Is it that we don't know of any other options? Or maybe we are not willing to make the necessary lifestyle changes to improve our health. Is it just easier to take a pill or pills? Is much of the increase in medication consumption a result of our unhealthy lifestyles—lack of sleep, poor nutrition, too much stress, and lack of movement? For many health issues, medications can be lifesavers. I just want to create awareness of the tremendous healing benefits that can occur with proper rest/recovery, nutrition, and movement/exercise, and give people more options when it comes to improving their health. Taking more medications may not always be the answer.

Over the past decade I have seen a steady rise in the number of medications people are taking. Whether it's reviewing a health history questionnaire from a personal training client, receiving an email from someone who has recently attended one of my seminars, or just talking to friends and family, *people are flat-out taking more medications than ever.* I am always curious as to how this medication process began. Did it start with a stomach medication to help with an occasional bout of acid reflux? Was the cholesterol level slowly creeping up? Was muscle and joint pain becoming more of a constant problem? Was getting a good night's sleep a thing of the past? Was the blood glucose too high? In most cases, people have said that the medication train started slowly, but quickly got out of control.

BONNIE'S JOURNEY

To get an idea how lifestyle choices can affect medication consumption, let me tell you a story about Bonnie Klinger and her journey to better health. Bonnie is sixty-three years old, a mother of two wonderful adult children, Rebecca and Steven, and has been married to her husband Jerry, the love of her life, for forty-five years. Bonnie has battled excess weight since she was a kid. She weighed 150 pounds when she was 11 years old, and her weight climbed to an all-time high of 207 pounds when she was in her late forties.

Bonnie defined "healthy" as being thin. In high school, Bonnie started eating one meal a day to lose enough weight to make the cheerleading squad, and she did. She kept riding an insidious on-again-off-again diet train for the next forty-five years. She tried just about every diet—fasting, low-fat, low-carb, no-carb, good-carb–bad-carb, low-calorie, high-fat, and a liquid meal-replacement diet.

Besides being overweight, Bonnie smoked two packs of cigarettes a day, seldom ate breakfast, ate lots of fast food, had a sedentary job, watched hours of television, and didn't do anything that could remotely be considered exercise. Bonnie's spirit had slowly been broken.

Then, over time, not only was Bonnie's spirit broken, her body started breaking down. She developed high blood pressure, hypothyroidism, osteoarthritis, allergies, high cholesterol, acid reflux, high triglycerides, low HDL, insulin resistance, and sleep apnea. Bonnie was up to ten prescription medications plus aspirin each day! Her cardiologist was planning to add even more medications and put her on a C-pap machine to aid her breathing while she slept.

Bonnie decided it was time to make some lifestyle changes. She started following a low-calorie diet and began exercising three times a week, and managed to lose nearly thirty pounds. She then hit a year-long plateau; she was no longer losing weight and was still taking eight prescription medications plus the aspirin. This was not Bonnie's vision of retirement!

In October 2005 Bonnie came to see me, and she was desperate to lose weight and get healthier. We started right from the beginning. I told Bonnie, "I want you to be healthy at the *cellular level*." I explained the basic foundation of *On Target Living Nutrition* and the *Food Target*. Bonnie thought she was in trouble when she looked at the *Food Target!* She did not like to eat fish, eggs, oatmeal, lentils, kale, collard greens, flax meal…or ostrich! She said, "Who eats ostrich?" I explained to Bonnie that to lose weight and get healthy changes have to occur at the cellular level, and she didn't have to eat ostrich!

Her current way of eating was making her unhealthy and weight loss was going to be extremely difficult to sustain. This was upsetting to Bonnie because she thought she was already making healthy choices. Bonnie was skeptical about many of the changes I recommended, especially eating every three hours and eating healthy fats. She thought, "Healthy fats? Whoever heard that fats can be healthy?" She thought she would gain weight eating this way.

I said to Bonnie, "Give me six weeks, and by the end of the year hopefully you can get off many of your medications." Normally when consulting with a client I start at a much slower pace, but Bonnie was desperate for change! She wanted to do everything in her power to be successful and wanted to dig in immediately! As Bonnie left my office I thought she was going to cry, so I tried to reassure her that everything was going to work out for the best. I said, "Let's take it one day at a time."

Bonnie went home and cleaned out her cupboards, refrigerator, and freezer of all processed foods. If the label read "partially hydrogenated" or "high-fructose corn syrup," out it went. She then went to the health food store and stocked her house with

flaxseed oil, cod liver oil, evening primrose oil, extra-virgin olive oil, extra-virgin coconut oil, rolled oats, venison, buffalo, organic dairy, chicken, fresh fruits, and vegetables. I told you she was on a mission! Bonnie and Jerry prepared all of their meals and snacks at home from these new foods and made healthier choices in restaurants. Bonnie met with her personal trainer, Rebecca Klinger, her daugh-

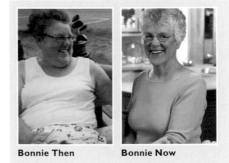

Bonnie Then   **Bonnie Now**

ter, who designed a program to fit Bonnie's goals and needs. She discussed what she was doing with her family physician and enlisted her support. Her physician encouraged her to keep track of her blood pressure and get blood work done after several weeks to monitor her response to her new exercise and nutritional changes.

After *only nine weeks* of *On Target Living Nutrition*, Bonnie had lost seventeen pounds. Her blood pressure, cholesterol, and triglycerides had improved so dramatically that her physician discontinued six of her medications and the daily aspirin.

Bonnie's health profile changes are truly amazing, but more amazing is what happened to her during this transformation—her smile, the excitement in her voice, her vitality, her soul. Bonnie virtually glows when you see her! She has become so passionate about helping others that she asked me if we could collaborate on writing a cookbook. She told me, "You know all this stuff about nutrition, but you don't know much about cooking!" The result is our new book, *On Target Living Cooking*.

MEDICATIONS CAN HELP

Medications can be extremely helpful and necessary in many situations. But we also need to give the body an opportunity to heal itself. The human body will try to heal itself if given enough time and the right ingredients. Why not give your body that opportunity?

Before accepting or using prescription medications, ask your physician a few tough questions:

1. Are there non-drug approaches that I can try first?
2. Exactly what condition is this medication supposed to treat?
3. What is my risk?
4. How much will this medication lower my risk?
5. What are the side effects of this medication?
6. Is it possible to eliminate this medication by making healthier food and exercise choices?

Now, don't run to the medicine cabinet and throw your medications down the drain. Remember, medications may play a role in leading a functional life, especially in the short run. Work closely with your physician and take an active role in your health. *Start slowly* by making healthier food and beverage choices, and think about what your medicine cabinet could look like in the future.

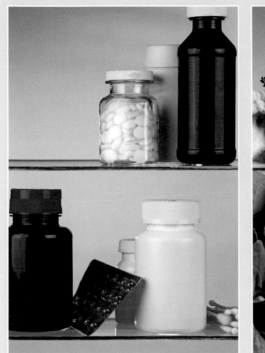
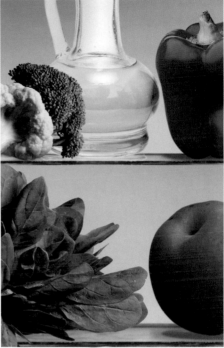

Typical medicine cabinet   Future medicine cabinet

THE BOTTOM LINE

1. America has become an overmedicated society.
2. The cost of prescription drugs is driving the cost of health care out of sight.
3. Each of us can take more responsibility for our own health.
4. Work closely with your physician and healthcare professionals.
5. Let food be your medicine!
6. Start by making small changes and develop these changes into daily habits.

TAKE IT FROM ME...

Having been one of those uncoordinated kids in school, hating PE and always picked last for any mandatory school team, I found all kinds of excuses not to exercise as an adult. I didn't like it, it was for people who cared about having a super attractive body to attract a mate, I didn't have time. You name it—I had an excuse. As a physician, I knew that this wasn't very wise, but also rationalized that my estrogen would protect me from the ravages of heart disease.

Janet Rose Osuch, MD

And eating! Well, I thought I was eating pretty well, when I did eat, which wasn't regularly. A typical menu? Coffee for breakfast. Lunch? Not having time to prepare a lunch before tearing out the door at 6:30 a.m. to begin my day, having few places to buy a decent lunch near my work, and being pressured to "work in" patients over the noon hour meant that I often ate lunch only when a colleague or I scheduled it over a work issue, or when I was so hungry I felt like I would faint if I didn't get something in my body soon. Typically, that might mean a candy bar. Ironically enough, during this time I counseled patients on the importance of a healthy lifestyle, including regular eating and exercising. But oh, I had a large low-fat meal consisting of lots of fruits and vegetables at night, to be sure! And I avoided fast-food restaurants as much as possible. How much healthier can you get?

My wake-up call for a lifestyle change came on February 27, 1998, when I was diagnosed with a benign brain tumor that was large enough to be causing symptoms requiring neurosurgical intervention. When I awoke from the post-operative coma ten days later, I weighed less than a hundred pounds. What little muscle I had had almost disappeared, and I couldn't walk. In fact, I couldn't even sit up straight in my wheelchair. My rehabilitation consisted of six hours a day, five days a week of intensive therapy for a month, followed by eight to ten hours per week of therapy over the next year. At the end of it, my physical rehabilitation therapist met with my new personal trainer, Chris Johnson, to help me transition between formal rehabilitation and personal training for one hour per week.

To my surprise, the first month that Chris and I met consisted mostly of nutritional counseling. I learned about all the eating mistakes that I was making and how to adopt eating habits that were to become life-long. The exercise regimen that he helped me establish has helped me understand that you don't need to be a professional athlete to care about your body and to help it function at an optimal level. The healthy lifestyle that I now lead has contributed enormously to my emotional well-being as well.

The contribution of Chris's mentoring, guidance, and caring has had a profound impact on my life. The circumstances of my need for his message are ones that I would not wish for any of you. I do, however, wish for each of you to be receptive to his message. It truly can change your life. It certainly changed mine.

Chapter 9
AIM FOR THE FOOD TARGET

USDA'S FOOD GUIDANCE—MY PYRAMID

Let's examine the differences between USDA's Food Guidance—MyPyramid—and the new *On Target Living Food Target*.

I understand the challenges of trying to come up with food guidelines for over 300 million people in the United States. I think most of the nutritional community across the country is in agreement that we need to exercise more, eat more fruits, vegetables, and whole grains,

> You really can change the world if you care enough.
>
> —Marian Wright Edelman

and drink more water. The USDA MyPyramid does a nice job recommending foods and serving sizes and emphasizing the need for regular exercise. But I believe that you, the consumer, need *more* information and more easily understandable information.

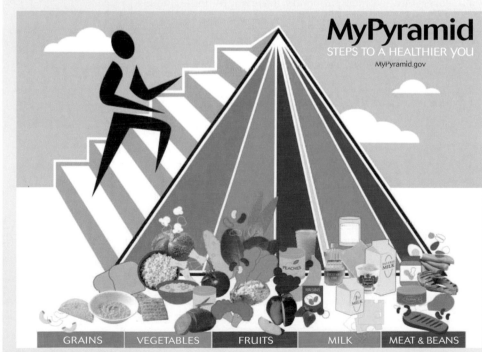

Source: U.S. department of agriculture/U.S. Department of Health and Human Services

The first shortcoming of the USDA MyPyramid is that it overlooks quality. The USDA MyPyramid gives little consideration to the source or quality of foods that we should or should not be eating. The USDA MyPyramid makes no distinction between healthy and unhealthy carbohydrates, proteins, and fats. But quality is everything when it comes to nutrition. Improving the quality of all your food and drink choices is one of the important concepts of *On Target Living Nutrition.*

The second shortcoming of the USDA MyPyramid is its recommendation about quantity. To begin with, the USDA MyPyramid recommends limiting your fat intake, so not enough quality fats are included. Consuming 20 to 35 percent of your calories from healthy fats is essential for optimal health and performance. Just as the recommendation for healthy fats is too low, the recommendation for milk consumption is too high. The USDA MyPyramid recommends the equivalent of at least three cups per day. Is this organic cow's milk, goat's milk, oat milk, rice milk, soy milk, or almond milk? If you enjoy milk, drink one or two cups a day and improve the quality of the milk you are drinking. What about your calcium needs if you only drink one or two cups of milk a day? Milk is not the only source of calcium. There are many other wonderful sources of calcium, such as broccoli, spinach, leafy greens, most vegetables, oatmeal, almonds, and fish, to name a few.

THE "TARGET MAN"

Over the past few years I have been working with Auto-Owners Insurance Company to help their workforce get healthier. Auto-Owners asked me if I would interview a few of their associates and then share their success stories with their entire organization. One gentleman I interviewed, Jim Fisher from Lakeland, Florida, told me how he had lost thirty-five pounds along with decreasing 75 percent of the medications he had been taking. Jim is sixty-six years old and full of life, and was proud to share his success and new lifestyle habits.

I asked Jim, "How did you do it?"

He said," I was not entirely clear on what to do, so I ate only the foods that were in the center of your *Food Target*," thus his new nickname "The Target Man."

I ended the interview by asking the most important question, "Why did you make the change?"

He said, "I was sixty-five years old, overweight, tired, and on too many medications, and my doctor said I was a borderline diabetic; it was time for a new life!"

Way to go, Jim.

The third shortcoming of the USDA MyPyramid is that it is confusing and assumes that people already know a great deal about food and beverages. I believe one of the greatest challenges in getting people to eat healthier is for them to understand food and beverage quality and then to learn how to slowly implement these changes. The USDA MyPyramid assumes the consumer understands the three macronutrients, food quality, and how to make incremental changes.

On Target Living Nutrition: FOOD TARGET

I suggest replacing the USDA MyPyramid with the On Target Living *Food Target* to guide your daily food choices. *The Food Target focuses on a balance of carbohydrates, proteins, and fats while incorporating an assessment of the quality of these nutrients.*

The new *Food Target* has the lowest nutritional value foods at the outside of the target. These are the foods that contribute the least nutrition to the body and can be detrimental to your health. In the *Food Target*, the most beneficial, most nutritious foods—those that make the body stronger—are closer to the center of the target. The idea behind the *On Target Living Nutrition* program is to achieve balanced eating around the target and to concentrate your eating as close to the center of the target as possible. These foods are in their most natural, unprocessed states. Most importantly, the *Food Target* allows people to change at their desired pace. They don't have to move from the outer ring to the center all at once! Place the *Food Target* on your refrigerator and refer to it on a daily basis. The *Food Target* can be found on the next page; a detachable version appears at the end of this book.

On Target Living Nutrition: **FOOD TARGET**

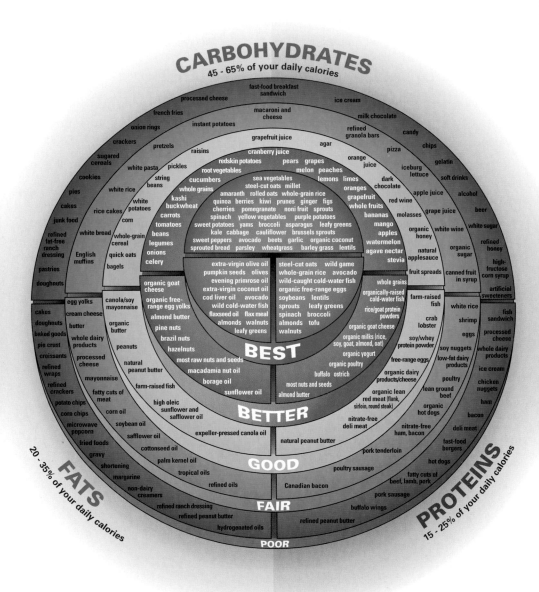

the core of
On Target Living
Nutrition

MACRONUTRIENTS:
THE CORE OF *On Target Living Nutrition*

What are macronutrients? Macronutrients are carbohydrates, proteins, and fats. Macronutrients are the fuel source for our bodies and minds.

- **Carbohydrates**—fuel your body

- **Proteins**—build your body

- **Fats**—heal your body

Learning to improve the quality of the foods you eat and the beverages you drink is the essence of the *On Target Living Nutrition* program. Use the *Food Target* as a learning tool and a lifelong guide for eating. The *Food Target* places the lowest-quality, most nutrient-deficient foods on the outer rings of the target, in the red area. These are the foods that are the least nourishing and can be detrimental to your health. The highest-quality, most nutrient dense foods—those that make the body stronger—are closer to the center of the *Food Target*, the green area. You will find unrefined whole foods closer to the center of the target.

Think about what you plan to eat. Is it a carbohydrate, protein, fat, or a combination of all three? Think about the quality of the foods. Do they belong along the outer rings of the *Food Target* or toward the center? Write down your food choices in a blank *Food Target* and analyze where they fall. Compare your *Food Target* with the sample *Food Target* to evaluate your selections. By using the *Food Target*, you learn to identify carbohydrates, proteins, and fats, and the quality of these macronutrients.

The idea behind the *On Target Living Nutrition* program is to achieve balanced eating around the target, concentrating your meals as closely as possible to the center of the target. Start slowly and make small changes.

Consuming quality macronutrients in balance is the core of *On Target Living Nutrition*. Throughout the next three chapters, I will help you understand how your waistline, energy, mood, overall day-to-day performance, and long-term health are affected by the quality and type of macronutrients you consume.

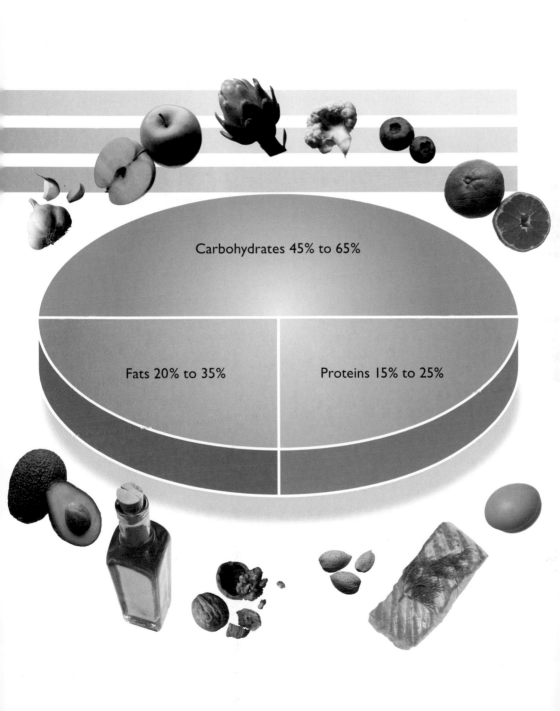

Carbohydrates 45% to 65%

Fats 20% to 35%

Proteins 15% to 25%

Chapter 10
FUEL YOUR BODY WITH CARBOHYDRATES

What is a carbohydrate? Carbohydrates are sugar chains linked together. Generally, the shorter the sugar chain, the more processed or refined the carbohydrate. The

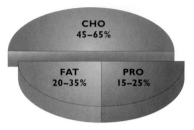

more refined or processed a carbohydrate, the less fiber, vitamins, minerals, phytochemicals, and antioxidants it contains. A longer sugar chain contains more fiber, vitamins, minerals, phytochemicals, and antioxidants. These are the types of carbohydrates that create better health and performance. Long-chain carbohydrates are whole foods with little or no refinement or processing. A doughnut and broccoli are both in the carbohydrate family, but that is where their similarity ends. Doughnuts have short sugar chains, are nutrient-deficient, and cause a quick spike in blood glucose. Broccoli, on the other hand, has long sugar chains, is nutrient-dense, and causes little change in blood glucose.

> The only people who never fail are those who never try.
>
> —Ilka Chase

Why do we need carbohydrates? Energy! *Carbohydrates are the body's main energy or fuel source.* Carbohydrates also provide the body with valuable fiber, vitamins, minerals, phytochemicals, and antioxidants for the brain and nervous system.

ARE CARBOHYDRATES HEALTHY OR UNHEALTHY?

I want to make it clear right from the beginning that carbohydrates are necessary for energy, health, and optimal performance. You will be reading a common phrase or question throughout the rest of this book: *it depends*. This phrase is critical to determine the quality of the foods or beverages you are consuming. So when someone asks whether carbohydrates are healthy or unhealthy, your answer is, "it depends!" *It depends on the quality of the carbohydrate.* A quality carbohydrate is one that delivers the most fiber, vitamins, minerals, phytochemicals, and antioxidants. Many people believe the best way to lose weight is to cut back on carbohydrate intake without fully understanding the role that high-quality carbohydrates play in keeping the body fit, healthy, and happy. With the growing demand for weight-loss diets, many carbohydrates have been lumped together as foods to avoid if you are trying to lose weight.

Not long ago I was approached by a woman in my hometown grocery store. She asked, "Aren't you that nutrition guy?"

I replied, "Yes, I have written a few books on nutrition and speak about nutrition in my seminars."

She asked, "Do you eat bananas?" I had a bunch of bananas in my grocery cart at the time. I said that yes, I ate bananas.

She then said, "I am a little surprised that you eat bananas. Did you know that they are high on the glycemic index?" I said that I knew that. She said, "I didn't think you would eat bananas due to their high glycemic index." She then started to walk away with a smirk on her face.

Caught off guard, I felt like I had just been scolded, and I think I was! I decided to walk after her. I could not let this go. "Excuse me," I said. "Since when did a banana become an unhealthy carbohydrate choice?" A banana is one of nature's perfect foods, beautifully packaged, full of vitamins, minerals, and fiber, and tastes great. She was not buying the benefits of eating a banana. In her mind bananas raise your blood glucose quickly and *make you fat!* Yes, bananas are high on the glycemic index, but because they have a high level of vitamins and minerals, they fall into the "better" category on the *Food Target*. You don't have to go through life being afraid of eating a banana or other fruits that are high in sugar. Enjoy the wonderful taste of eating a fresh piece of fruit and all the health benefits that they bring.

In many of the high-protein, low-carbohydrate diet plans, you take fruit out of your diet for the first few weeks, and many fruits are totally forbidden in the diet. Since when does a blueberry or an orange make you fat? To me this sends a message that fruit makes you fat. Yes, many processed carbohydrates contribute to poor health and weight gain, but we need a better understanding of all carbohydrates.

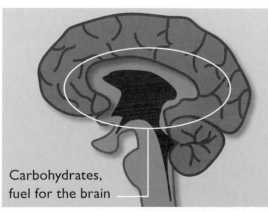

Carbohydrates, fuel for the brain

Carbohydrates are our energy foods. They are essential for better health and performance. Along with all the benefits mentioned earlier, carbohydrates are necessary to fuel the brain. The human brain needs 400 calories of carbohydrates per day to function properly. Carbohydrates are the only source of energy the brain can use, except during starvation.

Your goal each day should be to consume between 45 and 65 percent of your total calories from quality carbohydrates. Examples of carbohydrates include apples, asparagus, rolled oats, sweet potatoes, lentils, soda pop, and sugar. Some carbohydrates, such as cereals, bagels, and pasta, contain a large amount of carbohydrates. Other foods, such as leafy greens, asparagus, and broccoli, contain a small amount of carbohydrates.

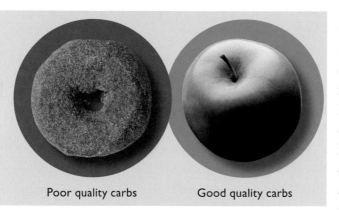

Poor quality carbs   Good quality carbs

In our fast-paced, convenient, prepackaged food society, carbohydrates fall on a continuum between refined and unrefined carbohydrates. Refined, lower-quality carbohydrates have been processed and stripped of essential nutrients and are lacking in fiber, vitamins, minerals, phytochemicals, and antioxidants. These include refined cereals, white bread, crackers, doughnuts, potato chips, candy, soda pop, instant potatoes, and sugar, to name a few. Unrefined, high-quality carbohydrates are foods in their most natural state. These include whole fruits, vegetables, whole grains, starches, and legumes. Consuming unrefined carbohydrates helps the body stay healthy and perform at its best. Carbohydrates are also our primary source of dietary fiber.

FIBER

Fiber is necessary for optimal health. Fiber helps reduce the risk of certain cancers, lowers cholesterol, stabilizes blood glucose and promotes regularity. Fiber absorbs water as it moves through the digestive tract and adds bulk to feces. Fiber moves food quickly through the digestive system and enhances fat loss. Fiber also slows down the insulin response. This is one reason that eating whole fruit does not raise your blood glucose as much as drinking fruit juice, which contains little or no fiber.

The National Cancer Institute recommends an intake of twenty-five to thirty grams of fiber daily. Most Americans eat less than fifteen grams per day!

Types of fiber

Water-soluble. Water-soluble fiber helps reduce cholesterol and slows insulin response. Some water-soluble fiber sources include steel-cut oats, rolled oats, oat bran, amaranth, millet, barley, beans, peas, and apples.

Water-insoluble. Water insoluble fiber helps supply the bulk that keeps food moving quickly through the digestive tract, acting like a broom sweeping out un-digested material, promoting regularity, and reducing the risk of certain kinds of cancers. Leafy greens, whole grains, root vegetables, and skins from fruits and vege-tables all contain water-insoluble fiber.

You can easily obtain twenty-five to thirty grams of fiber per day by eating foods in their most natural state, such as fruits, vegetables, whole grains, nuts, seeds, and beans.

While we are discussing fiber and its benefits, let's discuss the question, "How regular are you?" How often do you have a bowel movement?

Are you constipated more than you would like? The answer to this question in most cases is directly related to the quality of the food we eat and the beverages we drink or lack thereof. Some folks are like clockwork, same time, same place, you get the picture. Others are just the opposite. They have no regular pattern. They may go two days in a row and then do not have a bowel movement for three days. I have even had a few personal training clients tell me they have a bowel movement once or twice a week.

Having consistent bowel movements is one way to keep your body healthy. If your dog did not have a bowel movement for three days would you be concerned? Is my dog sick? Why is my dog constipated? Is my dog not getting enough water? Is my dog eat-ing the wrong type of food? You may want to ask yourself these same questions if you are not as regular as you would like.

A few years back I ruptured the patella tendon in my knee while playing basket-ball. It was an ugly injury, and I immediately went into surgery to get it repaired. After the surgery, the surgeon told me that in approximately three to four days I would be in a great deal of pain because the femoral block in my leg would be wearing off. I was given some strong pain medications to help with the pain and sent home.

The surgeon was right. At day three I was in a lot of pain, but it was not due to pain in my leg. It was from being constipated! I had not had a bowel movement in over three days! I had never taken prescription pain medications before, and one of the side effects of these medications is constipation. This was something new to me, and I was becoming desperate in my need to alleviate my discomfort. Due to my injury and surgery, I was highly medicated, dehydrated, and flat on my back, unable to move, and out of my normal eating patterns. I stopped taking my prescription pain medications and went to old reliable flax meal and flaxseed oil. Flaxseeds have been around for hundreds of years, and one of the benefits of using flax is that it keeps you regular. I tripled my normal dose, taking three tablespoons in the morning and three tablespoons in the afternoon and within an hour after the second dose my discomfort was gone. I was clean as a whistle. One question that comes up in my seminars occasionally is "what happens if you consume too much flax?" Now you know the answer!

There are many factors that contribute to regularity. Let constipation be a thing of the past by following a few simple tips:

1. Develop consistent meal patterns.

2. Eat more whole foods and high-quality fats.

3. Consume twenty-five to thirty grams of fiber per day.

4. Stay properly hydrated.

5. Get seven to eight hours of sleep each night.

6. Move your body on a daily basis.

Tips for adding more fiber to your diet

- Eat a big salad full of leafy greens daily.
- Sneak in vegetables whenever you can. Don't overcook as this decreases the fiber content.
- Eat more whole fruits. Berries, apples, and dried fruits are high in fiber.
- Eat more beans. Beans are loaded with fiber. A half cup of beans contains four to six grams of fiber.
- Eat whole grains instead of refined white versions. Look for whole-grain breads, pastas, and cereals.
- Bring on the nuts and seeds. Raw walnuts, almonds, flaxseeds, and flax meal are excellent sources of fiber.

Fiber grams per serving of various foods

Food		Food		Food	
garbanzo beans (½ cup)	8	oatmeal (½ cup)	4	spinach (3 oz.)	2
flax meal (3 tbs.)	6	potato (1 potato)	3	raisins (¼ cup)	2
whole-grain bread (1 slice)	6	green beans (1 cup)	3	white bread (1 slice)	1
broccoli (1 cup)	5	kale (3 oz.)	3	beef	0
apple (1 apple)	4	broccoli slaw (3 oz.)	3	chicken	0
blueberries (¾ cup)	4	walnuts (¼ cup)	3	tuna	0
raspberries (¾ cup)	4	almonds (¼ cup)	3		

TYPES OF CARBOHYDRATES

- **Fruits:** berries, oranges, apples, kiwi, cherries, prunes, figs, lemons, limes, grapefruit, watermelon, peaches, melon, pears, bananas, mangos, apricots, plums
- **Vegetables:** cauliflower, broccoli, asparagus, sweet peppers, kale, sprouts, cabbage, parsley, leafy greens, wheat grass, sea vegetables
- **Whole grains:** steel-cut oats, rolled oatmeal, millet, wheat, rye, amaranth, spelt, barley, quinoa, rice
- **Starches:** sweet potatoes, purple potatoes, redskin potatoes, squash, carrots, rutabagas, parsnips, beets
- **Legumes:** lentils, red beans, soybeans, chickpeas, navy beans, black beans, yellow or green peas

THE CARBOHYDRATE CONTINUUM

All sources of carbohydrates fall on a continuum between refined and unrefined. Your goal is to move to more unrefined sources of carbohydrates wherever possible. Consuming unrefined carbohydrates helps the body stay healthy and perform optimally.

Refined	The Carbohydrate Continuum	Unrefined
Fewer nutrients and fiber		More nutrients and fiber
white bread	enriched wheat bread	100% whole-grain bread
apple juice	natural applesauce	apple
catsup	organic catsup	tomato
sugared cereal	quick oats	100% rolled oats
corn syrup	creamed corn	whole-kernel corn
orange drink	100% orange juice	orange

CARBOHYDRATE CHEMISTRY

How carbohydrates work in the body

If you disliked chemistry in high school or college, this section may not be for you, so I will keep it fairly simple. Digestion breaks down the carbohydrates you consume into glucose. Digestion begins with the saliva in your mouth and continues through the stomach and intestines. As the carbohydrates are broken down, glucose passes into the bloodstream. The pancreas is the organ that controls blood glucose levels by unlocking two opposing hormones: *insulin* and *glucagon*.

When you eat, your blood glucose level begins to rise. In response to a rising blood glucose level, insulin is released to allow the cells to be fed. Insulin opens up the cells to allow blood glucose in. The cells then use glucose for energy, or store it as glycogen (carbohydrate) or fat. The cells call upon these stored nutrients when other nutrients are not available. When energy stores are full, excess blood glucose is stored as fat.

Insulin is the key that opens up your cells for nourishment. Without insulin, your cells would starve to death. Insulin is a fat-storing and hunger hormone. The ideal is to produce a sufficient amount of insulin and have your cells sensitive enough to open up easily. If you produce too much insulin in response to an increase in food intake (like the sumo wrestlers), your body will store the excess carbohydrates, proteins, and fats as body fat.

Insulin is the key that opens up your cells for nourishment. Without insulin, your cells would starve to death.

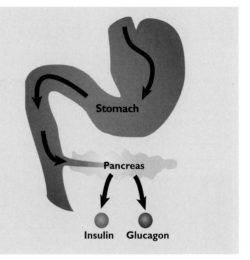

Stomach

Pancreas

Insulin   Glucagon

Insulin's opposing hormone is glucagon. Glucagon is the body's safety net in controlling blood glucose. It protects the body by preventing blood glucose from dropping too low. The pancreas releases glucagon as blood glucose drops. Glucagon directs the cells to release stored carbohydrate as glucose to raise your blood glucose level. Glucagon is a carbohydrate- and fat-releasing hormone.

Eating frequent small meals (150–400 calories per meal) throughout the day helps keep these hormones in balance. This is counter to the practice of many dieters, who stimulate their pancreas to overproduce insulin by eating one or two large meals per day.

THE GLYCEMIC INDEX

It can be difficult to predict how certain carbohydrates affect your blood glucose levels. Common sense would lead us to believe that most refined, processed carbohydrates cause a rapid rise in blood glucose and unrefined carbohydrates would have a smaller effect on blood glucose levels. In most cases this is true, but the accuracy of this method of determining how certain carbohydrates affect blood glucose can be greatly improved by using the glycemic index.

The glycemic index is a numeric tool that determines how individual carbohydrate foods affect blood glucose levels. Foods with a high glycemic index cause a large rise in blood glucose levels, and foods with a low glycemic index have a smaller impact on blood glucose levels. Five factors determine how quickly carbohydrates in a food break down into glucose and enter the bloodstream.

1. **The structure of the carbohydrate.** There are three types of sugar structures: glucose, fructose, and galactose. Glucose is found in grains, breads, pastas, cereals, vegetables, and starches. Fructose is found in fruit. Galactose is found in dairy products. Glucose is the only sugar structure that is released directly into the bloodstream. Fructose and galactose are absorbed first by the liver, which converts them to glucose, slowing down their release into the bloodstream. The sugar in rice cakes, bagels, and pasta enters the bloodstream very quickly, while the sugar in apples, pears, ice cream, and yogurt enters relatively slowly.

2. **How much the carbohydrate has been refined or processed.** Refined carbohydrates break down easily into glucose because they are stripped of valuable fiber. Then they quickly and easily enter the bloodstream. White bread has a high glycemic index as compared to whole-grain bread, in which the fiber is still intact. Grape juice has a much higher glycemic index than whole grapes.

3. **The fiber content of the carbohydrate.** Fiber slows down the release of carbohydrates into the bloodstream.

4. **Protein content of the food.** Protein slows the release of carbohydrates into the bloodstream.

5. **Fat content of the food.** Fat slows the release of carbohydrates into the bloodstream.

Glycemic index							
Foods rated 70 and above are high glycemic foods							
glucose	100	pretzels	83	watermelon	76		
cornflakes	92	rice cake	82	grape juice	75		
mashed potatoes	92	sugared cereal	81	bagel	72		
carrot	92	white bread	80	popcorn	72		
white rice	85	jelly beans	78	millet	71		
baked potato	85	doughnut	76	banana	70		
Foods rated 56–69 are moderate glycemic foods							
angel food cake	67	raisins	64	sweet corn	60		
whole-wheat bread	65	soft drink	63	white spaghetti	58		
cantaloupe	65	bran muffin	60	peas	57		
Foods rated 55 and below are low glycemic foods							
orange juice	52	yam	37	avocado	0		
brown rice	50	soy milk	36	leafy greens	0		
grapes	50	chickpeas	35	cucumber	0		
grapefruit juice	48	split peas	32	raw broccoli	0		
baked beans	48	lentils	29	walnuts	0		
skim milk	46	yogurt	28	almonds	0		
oatmeal (slow-cooking)	42	grapefruit	25	fish	0		
orange	42	tomato	19	egg	0		
rye bread	41	soybeans	18	chicken	0		
apple	40	green or red pepper	0				

Notice that the majority of foods at the high end of the glycemic index are refined foods and at the low end most of the foods have little refinement and are in their most natural state. Try to choose foods in their most natural state. Avoid refined carbohydrates that, in addition to being high on the glycemic index, may be high in sugar and low in fiber, vitamins, and minerals. If you do eat a food that is high on the glycemic index, balance these foods by eating some fats or proteins, which can slow the breakdown of the carbohydrate into glucose, and thereby slows its entrance into the bloodstream. Good examples are bananas and bagels. Using a banana in a smoothie made with protein and fat or eating a bagel with natural peanut butter slows the breakdown of these high-glycemic carbohydrates.

The *amount* of carbohydrate also affects your blood glucose. Eating a half cup of carrots is going to have a much smaller impact on your blood glucose levels than eating a half cup of raisins. Carrots have a higher rating than raisins on the glycemic index (ninety-two to sixty-four), but the amount of calories from a half cup of cooked carrots is 50 and the amount of calories from half cup of raisins is 230. It is important to understand the glycemic index in conjunction with the number of calories you consume. We will discuss more about quantity in Chapter 21.

WHY DO WE CRAVE CARBOHYDRATES?
The carbohydrate black hole

After eating too many or the wrong carbohydrates at one time, blood glucose will rise rapidly, creating an insulin overshoot in which the body releases more insulin than is needed. Blood glucose skyrockets. You get this great satisfaction for a short period of time before the bottom drops out and your energy plummets, creating a strong desire to raise your blood glucose again or take a nap! Have you ever overindulged by eating too many refined, low-quality carbohydrates like chips, crackers, stuffing, mashed potatoes, cookies, or ice cream? How did you feel?

A few years ago I found myself in the *carbohydrate black hole* on Christmas day by consuming seventeen, yes seventeen, Christmas cookies! My wife, Paula, makes these wonderful-tasting date cookies, and I told myself that I would have just one! My first mistake was thinking I was going to be able to eat just one. My second mistake was that I started eating these cookies on an empty stomach. Then one went to three and by the end of the night I think I consumed seventeen cookies! The entire day I felt lethargic and tired, as though I had been drugged, and the truth of the matter: I *was* drugged. I had a sugar hangover, and I felt lousy.

Once you start down this path of eating these unhealthy carbohydrate sources, it becomes extremely difficult to get out of this black hole. Occasionally, we all may enter into the carbohydrate black hole. Getting there can be fun, but once we arrive the fun is gone.

As a personal trainer I see this with many clients. They complain of low energy and the need for a quick picker-upper to increase their energy. When I look at their food logs, I see too many refined carbohydrates (those foods in the red area of the *Food Target*), little

The Black Hole

Once we get in,
can we ever get out?

protein, and virtually no healthy fats. People experience highs and lows as their energy levels rise and fall due to their consumption of refined carbohydrates and the overproduction of insulin that results. Most Americans try to control their energy with refined carbohydrates or with caffeine in a soft drink or coffee.

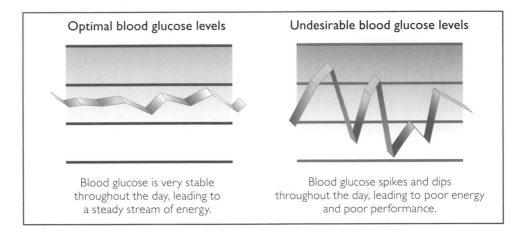

Optimal blood glucose levels	Undesirable blood glucose levels
Blood glucose is very stable throughout the day, leading to a steady stream of energy.	Blood glucose spikes and dips throughout the day, leading to poor energy and poor performance.

Insulin is a hunger hormone

Insulin is a powerful hunger hormone that triggers humans to eat. Once insulin is overproduced by eating too much or the wrong types of carbohydrates (red area on the *Food Target*), insulin becomes a powerful hunger trigger.

Thanksgiving gives us a perfect example of how insulin works as a hunger trigger. The average American consumes 2,000 to 4,000 calories at a single meal on Thanksgiving. Within a short time, the nap syndrome kicks in, just as with the sumo wrestlers, who promptly go to sleep following their single big meal of the day. Upon waking, your first urge is to eat again. You probably are not craving that leftover broccoli. No, you most likely want a sandwich with lots of bread, mashed potatoes, stuffing, or another piece of pie. This is the effect of the hunger hormone, insulin. As insulin levels rise to extreme heights after a very large meal, blood glucose will drop quickly, creating hunger for more refined carbohydrates.

Carbohydrates as mood regulators

When we become stressed or have low mood levels, we instinctively reach for comfort foods, which are often refined starchy carbohydrates. Eating refined starchy carbohydrates, those in the red area of the *Food Target*, elevates blood glucose too quickly along with increasing activity of serotonin. Serotonin is a neurotransmitter used by the brain for communication. Serotonin has a calming effect on the brain. Even though refined carbohydrates increase serotonin activity and make you feel good, this good feeling is only temporary, due to the spike in blood glucose and the ensuing drop in energy. This is one reason I consume whole grains such as oatmeal in the morning, sweet potatoes and one slice of whole-grain sprouted bread in the evening. These unrefined carbohydrates, those in the green area of the *Food Target*, also increase serotonin activity, but keep my brain happy and my energy high for a sustained period of time.

THE LOWDOWN ON SWEET STUFF

We are also a nation that likes our sweets for comfort foods. What if your comfort food is a refined sweet carbohydrate like cake, cookies, ice cream, candy, or regular soda pop? How does your body react to sweet carbohydrates? The same as with a refined starchy carbohydrate: little nutrient value, just calories!

More and more people are asking whether there are more healthy options available than refined sugar or chemically based sugar substitutes. I am going to keep this section short and simple. Instead of getting into explaining all the problems with artificial sweeteners or the benefits of using other sugar substitutes, I am going to give you my short list of higher-quality, healthier alternatives: *Stevia, agave nectar, organic cane sugar, organic honey,* and *organic molasses.* Stevia and agave nectar have little effect on blood glucose. Organic cane sugar, organic honey, and organic molasses each are quickly absorbed in the body, raising blood glucose quickly.

Stevia

Let's begin with stevia. Stevia is made from *Stevia rebaudiana,* a small shrub native to Paraguay in South America. Stevia was first discovered in 1887 by a South American nature scientist by the name of Antonio Bertoni. In its natural state, the stevia herb is ten to fifteen times sweeter than sugar. Stevia extracts can range anywhere from 100 to 300 times sweeter than sugar. My favorite powdered extract is Stevia Plus™. The equivalent of Stevia Plus™ to sugar is ¼ teaspoon Stevia Plus™ to one teaspoon of sugar. Stevia Plus™ has no calories.

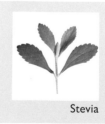

Stevia

For over fifty years, stevia has been used in Japan, and today stevia is being used around the world. The safety record for stevia usage is truly amazing. With the massive quantities of stevia and stevia extracts that are consumed each year, there have been no known cases of stevia overdoses or toxicity to humans reported during the past forty years. Stevia is also one sweetener people suffering from yeast-type conditions such as *Candida* can tolerate.

How does stevia taste? Personally, I like the taste of Stevia Plus™. I sometimes use it in a smoothie drink or in a recipe that calls for sugar, but it does have a different flavor from sugar. Many of my personal training clients say that they truly like the flavor, but it did take a little getting used to. Stevia does not break down when it is heated, so it can be used in baking or cooking. Stevia can be found in your local natural food stores and is now in many traditional grocery stores and supermarkets.

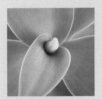

Agave nectar

Agave nectar

Agave nectar is a natural sweetener made from the juice of the agave plant. Agave nectar has a nice flavor, has the consistency of honey, and is suitable for all of your sweetening needs. Agave nectar can be found in your local natural food stores.

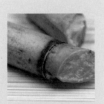

Organic cane sugar

Organic cane sugar

Most of the white sugar that is so common in the United States is highly refined by chemical processes from sugar cane, corn, or beet sugar. If your want the real deal, then look no further than organic cane sugar. It looks like sugar and tastes like sugar, without the chemical processing. Organic cane sugar can be found in many traditional grocery stores and most natural food stores.

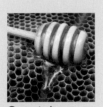

Organic honey

Organic honey

Honey has been around for centuries, most likely due to its wonderful texture and taste. I love the taste of a honey on a warm piece of whole-grain toast. Many people believe honey has many health benefits. The truth is that honey does contain small amounts of enzymes and minerals that sugar does not have. However, bees are subject to a variety of illnesses, which is one reason why it is not recommended to give honey to children under the age of two. The best source of honey is what you can buy from a local source, has not been heated to temperatures over 105 degrees, and is slightly cloudy. Too much heat and filtration destroy some of the beneficial properties of honey. Use honey on your cereal, a piece of toast, in your favorite recipe, or in a cup of hot tea and enjoy its wonderful flavor!

Organic molasses

Molasses is thicker than honey and has a strong flavor. Molasses, especially blackstrap molasses, has more minerals than any other sweetener. Blackstrap molasses is rich in iron, calcium, and potassium. Molasses is also the most alkaline of all sweeteners. It is not sensitive to heat, making it an excellent choice for baking. Your best choice is organic dark molasses.

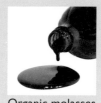
Organic molasses

HOW MANY CARBOHYDRATES SHOULD YOU EAT EACH DAY?

Carbohydrates are essential for optimal health and well-being. Choose carbohydrates in their most natural state, those that lie in the green areas of the *Food Target*. Your goal should be to get 45 to 65 percent of your calories from high-quality, unrefined carbohydrates. See the guide below for carbohydrate intake compared to overall calorie intake.

Recommended carbohydrate consumption based on daily calorie intake		
Total calories	Grams of carbohydrates	Number of carbohydrate calories
1,200	135–195	540–780
1,500	170–245	675–975
1,800	200–290	810–1,170
2,000	225–325	900–1,300
2,500	280–405	1,125–1625
3,000	335–485	1,350–1950

THE BOTTOM LINE

1. Carbohydrates are your body's main energy source. Forty-five to sixty-five percent of your daily food intake should come from quality carbohydrate sources, those in the green areas of the *Food Target*.

2. Carbohydrates are sugar chains linked together. Some, like soda pop, include short sugar chains (red area of the *Food Target*), while others, including broccoli, have long sugar chains (green area of the *Food Target*).

3. The National Cancer Institute recommends twenty-five to thirty grams of fiber per day.

4. Stevia and agave nectar are excellent sugar substitutes that do not elevate blood glucose and are easily tolerable for those who suffer from yeast-type conditions.

5. The carbohydrate black hole occurs when you eat too much food at one time or too many processed carbohydrates, raising blood glucose too rapidly followed by a severe drop in blood glucose and low energy.

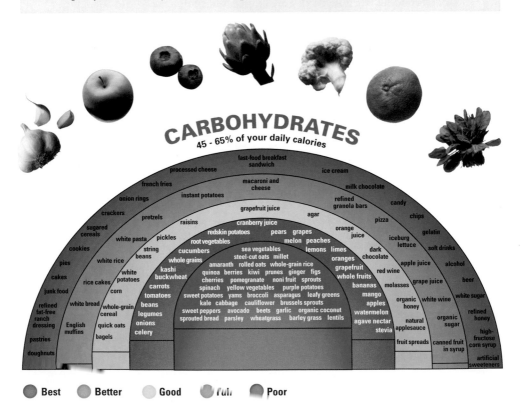

CARBOHYDRATES
45 - 65% of your daily calories

Best   Better   Good   Fair   Poor

Chapter 11
BUILD YOUR BODY WITH PROTEIN

The word *protein* comes from the Greek word *proteins*, which means "of prime importance." Protein is essential to life! Protein plays a role in every cell of the body. Proteins create hormones, maintain the immune system, build muscle, transport vitamins, and main-

> You create your own universe as you go along.
>
> —Winston Churchill

tain our blood, skin, and connective tissue. We all need to consider the **quality, quantity,** and the **frequency** with which we eat protein.

WHAT IS PROTEIN?

Our bodies break down protein into smaller nitrogen-containing units called amino acids. There are twenty-two amino acids: nine essential amino acids and thirteen non-essential amino acids. The body cannot manufacture essential amino acids, so we must get them through the foods we eat. If any of the essential amino acids is missing from our diet, a protein deficiency will develop.

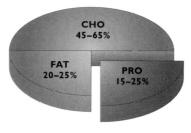

Complete and incomplete proteins

Complete proteins contain all nine essential amino acids. Sources of complete protein include eggs, meat, dairy products, poultry, fish, soy, and most nuts.

Incomplete proteins include some, but not all, of the essential amino acids. Foods that contain incomplete proteins include grains, rice, vegetables, and beans. It is relatively easy to get all of your essential amino acids from incomplete protein sources if you are eating a variety of *whole food sources.*

When eaten together the following combinations of incomplete proteins make complete proteins that are easily absorbed into the body:

- corn and beans
- rice and lentils
- peanut butter sandwich on whole-grain bread
- vegetable/tofu stir-fry

- oatmeal with almonds, hazelnuts, rice, or soy milk
- vegetarian chili with beans
- bean soup and whole-grain bread

BENEFITS OF PROTEIN

In addition to keeping the body strong and healthy, eating high-quality protein has further benefits:

Cell Development. Protein ensures that your body receives appropriate amounts of the essential amino acids for cell development. This includes connective tissue, skeletal muscle, skin, hair, and nails.

Increased Energy. Protein increases your energy level almost overnight! Having a stable blood glucose level is the name of the game in maintaining a high energy level throughout the day. Protein helps stabilize your blood glucose level. If your blood glucose is stable, insulin will not be overproduced, leaving you with greater energy. It is as easy as adding a piece of salmon to your favorite salad for lunch or adding a few nuts to your cereal in the morning. This will help stabilize your blood glucose and help maintain that much-needed energy required for you to feel your best!

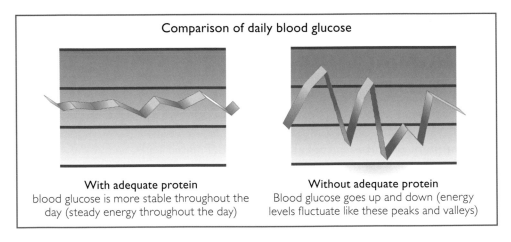

Comparison of daily blood glucose

With adequate protein
blood glucose is more stable throughout the day (steady energy throughout the day)

Without adequate protein
Blood glucose goes up and down (energy levels fluctuate like these peaks and valleys)

Reduced cravings for refined carbohydrates. By adding protein to your daily diet, your cravings for carbohydrates, especially the refined carbohydrates in the red area of the *Food Target*, will diminish.

Glucagon stimulation. Glucagon is insulin's opposing hormone. Insulin is a fat- and carbohydrate-storing hormone. Glucagon is a fat- and carbohydrate-releasing hormone that aids in stabilizing blood glucose and boosting metabolism. Protein helps to stimulate glucagon.

Improved brain power. Adequate amounts of protein can improve cognitive skills, memory, focus, and alertness. The first brain function to suffer the effects of age is memory. Memory begins to decline at about age thirty and loss of memory accelerates after age forty. To prevent this decline in memory and improve cognitive skills, focus, and alertness, all nine essential amino acids must be consumed daily in adequate amounts.

WHAT KINDS OF PROTEIN SHOULD YOU EAT?

If you asked most people in the United States the first thing that comes to their minds when they hear the word protein, I believe the answer would be meat, eggs, or dairy products, proteins that come from animal sources. For years we have focused our attention on animal sources of protein to reach our protein requirements. We need to understand that a great deal of our daily protein can and should come from plant sources.

During one of my seminars, a member of the audience asked me what I ate for breakfast. I said that a typical breakfast for me consisted of organic rolled oats, slivered almonds, dried organic cherries, soy milk, lemon-flavored cod liver oil, flaxseed oil, and a dash of cinnamon. I mix all the ingredients together and let it sit in the refrigerator overnight, no cooking required! I call this "oatmeal on the run." I love the taste; it is quick and easy, well-balanced, high in quality, and gives me great energy

CJ's breakfast

⅓ cup organic rolled oats: 8 grams of protein
slivered almonds: 5 grams of protein
I cup organic soy milk: 5 grams of protein
organic dried cherries: I gram of protein
cod liver oil: 0 grams of protein
flaxseed oil: 0 grams of protein
dash of cinnamon: 0 grams of protein
Total protein: I9 grams

to start my day. The member of the audience asked, "Where is your protein? Your breakfast seems low in protein."

So I said, "Let's take a closer look and see if this breakfast is low in protein."

I think many people were surprised by the amount of protein! This breakfast is just one example of high-quality protein from plant-based sources.

The protein debate

There is a growing debate over the best source of protein for the human body— animal or plant. From an environmental standpoint, eating plant-based protein is a great deal more efficient for our environment. It takes over fifty grams of grain to make one gram of protein from beef, without even considering the environmental effects of waste material from our animals. I am not a vegetarian. I enjoy many sources of animal proteins, but I want you to understand that plant sources of protein are not only good for our environment, they are also good for the human body. The real question is how can you improve the *quality* of your protein sources, whether it comes from an animal or plant?

> Choose pesticide-, growth hormone-, and antibiotic-free organic animal sources of protein whenever possible.

If you choose to consume animal-based protein sources, try to move to more organic sources. Why? The quality of our animal proteins is not what it used to be. In this age of growth hormones, antibiotics, pesticides, and synthetic fertilizers, the quality of our animal proteins has changed. Organic animal sources of protein look and taste better, and are healthier for the human body. For example, when comparing eggs from an organically raised chicken to a non-organically raised chicken, the organically raised chicken wins hands down. The eggshell is harder, the egg yolk is brighter in color, and the egg is much more flavorful.

Eggs

When most people think of eggs, their first thought is that eggs are high in cholesterol and that eating eggs may cause heart disease. Yes, an egg yolk does contain 200 mg of cholesterol. For some people, a high intake of cholesterol directly affects the amount of cholesterol in the bloodstream. But let's clear up a few misconceptions about eggs. First, the egg white itself is free of fat. Each egg white contains six grams of complete protein. The egg yolk is low in saturated fat and contains many other nutrients that are good for you, such as vitamins E and B, folic acid, choline (needed for proper brain functioning), and lecithin. Lecithin acts as a cholesterol-lowering agent and a natural emulsifier, helping prevent plaque buildup from blocking arteries. Eggs are also inexpensive and easy to prepare.

When buying eggs, your first choice should be organic free-range or cage-free eggs. Organic free-range eggs come from chickens raised in healthier environments, creating a healthier egg. Consume egg yolks in moderation, one or two per day. Eggs can fit nicely into a diet for people who enjoy them.

I like to eat eggs on a regular basis. I use one tablespoon of organic extra-virgin coconut oil and scramble four or five egg whites and one yolk, add a piece of fruit or vegetables, and in just four to five minutes I have an easy, balanced, great-tasting meal!

Fish

Fish is a high-protein food that provides a range of health benefits. White-fleshed fish are lower in fat than any other source of animal protein, and fish high in oils contain substantial quantities of healthy omega-3 fats. Though generally a good source of protein, *not all fish are created equal.* Just as the quality of our animal proteins is changing, the same can be said of the fish we eat. Most of the fish consumed in the United States today is farm raised. Ninety-five percent of all salmon consumed today in the United States is farm raised. Is farm-raised fish good for you? My answer is, *it depends!* It depends on the environment and what the fish are being fed; these two factors determine how good the fish is for you. Our rivers, lakes, and oceans are slowly becoming more polluted, and the fish living in these environments are becoming more toxic. Women who are pregnant should avoid consuming fish such as bluefin tuna, grouper, swordfish, marlin, orange roughy, and Chilean seabass due to its high mercury content.

Farm-raised fish are the future of our fish industry, whether we like it or not. We are starting to see an increase in the quality of farm raising fish practices, similar to the methods being used today in raising organic animals. If you have an opportunity to eat wild Alaskan salmon or rainbow trout caught from a stream in the mountains of Colorado, thank your lucky stars and enjoy the great taste and wonderful health benefits. If you don't have access to these fish grown in the wild, then farm-raised fish can be a good source of protein, especially if purchased from a high-quality fish farm. The wonderful benefits of fish oils will be discussed in greater detail in the next chapter.

Best Seafood Choices		
Abalone	*Herring, Atlantic	Shrimp, northern
*Anchovies	*Mackerel, Atlantic	Shrimp, Oregon pink
Arctic char	Mahimahi, Atlantic	Shrimp
Catfish	Mussels	Spot prawns
Caviar	*Oysters	Striped bass
Clams	*Sablefish/black cod	Sturgeon
Crab, dungeness	*Salmon, wild	Tilapia
Crab, snow	*Salmon, canned pink/ sockeye	*Tuna, albacore (canned white)
Crawfish	*Sardines	*Tuna, Skipjack (canned light)
Halibut, Pacific	Scallops	

*Indicates fish that are high in omega-3 fatty acids and low in environmental contaminants.

Poultry

Chicken: As when choosing eggs, your best choice is organic, free-range chicken.

Turkey: Turkey is much lower in saturated fat than most red meat. Like red meat, it is available in many forms—whole, or in parts, for roasting or baking, sliced for grilling, or ground as a delicious, healthy substitute for hamburger in soups, stews, pasta sauce, casseroles, and your other favorite recipes.

Ostrich: Ostrich is becoming a popular alternative to both red meat and other forms of poultry. It is low in saturated fat and high in protein, and is typically served as ostrich steaks or burgers or in soups. Ostrich is great for grilling and has excellent flavor.

Lean red meat

Most red meat contains high levels of unhealthy saturated fats that may lead to many health problems. However, choosing a higher-quality source of red meat can be part of a

Lean red meat choices		
Beef	Venison	Goat
Lamb	Elk	
Buffalo	Veal	

healthy, balanced diet and is a good source of iron. Grass-fed/organic is best when choosing red meat.

Throw a buffalo roast in a crock pot with a bunch of root vegetables on a cool autumn day. Yum!

The other white meat

Pork, along with red meat, may contain high levels of unhealthy saturated fat. Choose lean cuts of pork such as pork tenderloin or lean pork chops.

Dairy products

If you enjoy dairy products such as cow's milk, cottage cheese, yogurt, cheese, or butter, choose 100-percent organic sources whenever possible.

Many people are or may be allergic to the lactose found in cow's milk and are looking for alternatives. There are many milk options that taste great and are plant-based and lactose-free. These include oat, multi-grain, soy, rice, hazelnut, and almond milk, to name a few.

Another option to traditional cow's milk is goat's milk. Goat's milk is the most widely consumed dairy beverage in the world. Sixty-five percent of the world's population consumes goat's milk. Those who have digestion problems may truly benefit. Goat's milk is generally easy to digest and absorb due to the small size of its protein molecule. Whereas cow's milk requires up to two or three hours of digestion and absorption, goat's milk requires only twenty to thirty minutes!

There are multiple choices when choosing dairy products. Choose organic, high-quality, low-fat dairy products in moderation.

Plant-based proteins

Just like the breakfast example I used earlier in this chapter, I still think many people are confused over plant-based proteins. I have had numerous questions about the *Food Target* as to whether a food is a carbohydrate, a protein, or a fat. I have to explain that most foods have a mixture of the three macronutrients. For example, broccoli, which is a vegetable and is part of the carbohydrate family, also contains protein. In fact, one cup of broccoli contains four grams of protein, containing over 40 percent of its calories by weight. Here are a few other examples of plant-based proteins:

Plant-based proteins	
Steel-cut oats (½ cup): 12 grams of protein	Natural peanut butter (1 tablespoon): 5 grams of protein
Rolled oats (½ cup): 6 grams of protein	Walnuts (1 ounce): 4 grams of protein
Kidney beans (½ cup): 7 grams of protein	Peas (½ cup): 5 grams of protein
Soybeans (½ cup): 10 grams of protein	Baked yams: 4 grams of protein
Soy milk (1 cup): 7 grams protein	Raisins (¼ cup): 1 gram of protein
Whole-grain bread (1 slice): 6 grams of protein	Banana: 1 gram of protein
Almonds (1 ounce): 6 grams of protein	

The next time you are looking for high-quality protein sources, don't forget your plant-based protein sources.

Protein supplements

If you are following a vegetarian diet or are just plain busy, protein supplements can be a beneficial, quick, and easy addition to help balance your diet. There are many types of protein supplements to choose from: hemp, rice, soy, goat, whey, egg, and milk protein isolates. Most protein supplements come in a powder form. There has been some debate over which protein supplements are best.

Hemp. Hemp is my first choice when choosing a protein supplement. Hemp contains all essential amino acids, is more alkaline; is high in fiber, chlorophyll, magnesium, zinc, and iron; and is easy to digest. Hempseed is one of nature's superfoods.

Rice. Rice is an excellent source of plant-based protein, is inexpensive, absorbs easily, mixes well, and has a mild flavor.

Soy. Soy is a good source of plant-based protein, is easy to mix, and has a mild flavor. Some soy-based protein sources may be genetically modified or processed with hexane. *Choose only non–genetically modified and hexane-free food sources!*

Goatein. Goatein is my first choice when choosing an animal-based protein supplement. Goatein is made from goat's milk, is easily digestible, mixes well, and inhibits *Candida,* a fungus that inhabits the intestinal tract and mucous membranes of every living person. If the immune system is compromised when friendly bacteria in the gut are killed by taking antibiotics, a *Candida* infection may quickly follow. Goatein is an excellent source of protein for those who may be allergic to or have problems digesting other protein supplements. Goatein has a strong flavor, but that can be easily masked by adding your favorite fruit in a smoothie beverage.

Whey. Whey is derived from cow's milk. Whey is low in lactose, easy to mix, and has a mild flavor.

Egg albumin. Egg protein powder is not as popular as some of the other protein sources due to its strong flavor, and it does not mix well, but it can be an excellent source of protein.

Milk protein isolates. Similar to egg, milk protein isolates are not as popular as some of the other protein supplements due to flavor and ease of mixing. Milk protein isolates, unlike whey, are high in lactose.

How to choose a protein supplement:

1. **Plant- or animal-based protein:** Do you want a plant- or animal-based protein supplement?
2. **Short ingredients list:** The shorter the ingredients list the better.
3. **Highest quality of ingredients:** The quality of the protein supplement depends on the quality of ingredients. Choose only high-quality ingredients.
4. **Choose organic:** Whenever possible choose organic protein supplements.
5. **Ease of digestion:** Many people have difficulty digesting and absorbing certain protein supplements. There are many choices. Don't give up on the first one you try.

How to use protein supplements

One complaint I get from many of my personal training clients and seminar attendees is that it is challenging to eat frequently and that getting protein throughout the day can be difficult. It can be challenging to find time to eat and especially to get a balance of protein with each meal or snack. This is where a smoothie drink containing a balance of high-quality proteins, fats, and carbohydrates may come in. Instead of reaching for a prepackaged meal-replacement drink, a candy bar, a bag of chips from the vending machine, or a quick trip to the fast-food drive-through, make your own high-quality, healthy, balanced smoothie. I make up my smoothie the night before, using frozen berries, banana, water, flax meal, and hemp protein powder. This allows me to eat frequently, keep my energy high throughout the day, and get the balance of carbohydrates, proteins, and fats I need to keep my body strong and healthy. Oh, I almost forgot, it also tastes good!

A few years back one of my personal training clients was complaining of having low energy late in the afternoon. I recommended that he eat a balanced snack in the afternoon to maintain his energy level. At the age of seventy-five, full of passion, and the CEO of his company, he thought this was a great idea, but felt it may be difficult to eat a balanced snack due to his meeting schedule. So I suggested making up a balanced smoothie the night before and using this as his afternoon snack. "Great," he said, "I will start this tomorrow."

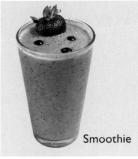

Smoothie

The following week we met again, and he had this weird look on his face. I said, "How are you doing? Did the balanced smoothie improve your energy?"

He said, "NO!" Then he proceeded to tell me that his smoothie was the nastiest-tasting drink he had ever tried.

I said, "Your smoothie did not taste good?"

He said, "It was awful; nobody should ever have to drink something that bad."

"Okay," I said, "tell me exactly how you made your smoothie."

He said, "I did exactly what you told me, one banana, sixteen ounces of frozen berries, three cups of water, two tablespoons of flax meal, and *three cups of protein powder.*"

I said, "You added three cups of protein powder? I said, 'three *ounces* of protein powder, not three cups.'"

He said, "It was like trying to drink mud."

I said, "It *was* mud." We had a great laugh over this. He tried the real recipe and his energy improved greatly. He also liked the taste.

The moral to this story: your food and beverage choices do not have to taste bad to be good for you. Experiment with your food and beverage choices. If they are not exactly what you are looking for, keep trying.

Protein/energy bars

Many varieties of protein or energy bars are available in the market today. I believe the quality of many of the new bars coming into the market has greatly improved. Many bar manufacturers now use high-quality whole food and organic ingredients in their bars and have improved the taste. Like the smoothies, protein/energy bars can be beneficial as a quick and easy snack when traveling or simply when you have a busy schedule and need some nourishment on the run. I caution my personal training clients against using these bars as meal replacements on a regular basis. Don't get caught up in the idea that they can or should replace quality whole foods every day!

Recently a health club member asked me, "What is that ugly greenish-brown thing you are eating?"

I replied, "It is an organic protein/energy bar."

He said, "That looks awful!"

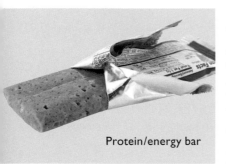

Protein/energy bar

I said, "It may not look so good, but it actually tastes great." I don't have much credibility when it comes to my opinion on something tasting good. Then I explained how healthy it was, and that it has high-quality ingredients, contained healthy fats, and was balanced. You name it, I was trying to sell him on why I was eating it. I don't think he was buying any of it. I don't think he could get out of his mind how anyone could eat something that looked that bad. So I said to him, "Try a piece and see what you think." He actually ate a piece after much begging on my part. It was like Mikey on that old Life Cereal commercial, he liked it! Two days later I saw him eating one of those bars as he was walking out of the club!

When choosing a protein/energy bar many people make the mistake of first looking at the total number of calories in the bar. Second, they look at the number of protein grams in relationship to the carbohydrate and fat grams. They believe that if the bar is high in protein and low in carbohydrates and fat, it must be a good choice! Remember, getting adequate, high-quality protein in your diet is important, but high-quality carbohydrates and fats are also important. When choosing a protein/energy bar, be sure to read the label and pay close attention to four considerations:

1. **Number of ingredients:** A good rule of thumb: the fewer ingredients, the better.
2. **Quality of ingredients:** Choose bars with the highest-quality ingredients. If you cannot pronounce a word in the ingredient list, then you probably don't want to put it in your body! Many bars now contain organic, high-quality ingredients. Avoid bars with fractionated or partially hydrogenated oils and those that contain high-fructose corn syrup.
3. **Balance:** Choose a bar that is balanced with high-quality carbohydrates, proteins, and fats.
4. **Taste:** You can have your cake and eat it too when it comes to taste! Just because a protein/energy bar is healthy for you does not mean it has to taste yucky! There are many bars that fit into the category of healthy for you along with great taste.

TAKE IT FROM ME...

Chris Johnson has been my health mentor for over ten years. He has extensive education about health and eating, stays current, and has many years of experience working with thousands of people on proper nutrition and exercise. He changes people's lives. His philosophies come out clearly in an easy-to-read style and show that diets don't work and eating healthy is not a sacrifice.

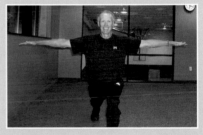

Al Arens

On Target Living Nutrition is the foundation of my health goals. My health goals are twofold: to be healthy and active for as long as possible and to be a role model for healthy living to my children, grandchildren, and friends. I get all of the information I need for these goals from *On Target Living Nutrition*.

My wife and I give *On Target Living Nutrition* as gifts to our children, grandchildren, and friends. Their gift to us is taking care of their health. The *Food Target* is placed prominently in our kitchen and is worth the price of the book by itself.

THE PROTEIN CONTINUUM

All sources of protein fall on a continuum between refined and unrefined. Your goal is to move to more unrefined sources of protein whenever possible. Consuming unrefined proteins helps the body stay healthy and perform optimally.

	The Protein Continuum	
Refined		Unrefined

Fewer nutrients and fiber			More nutrients and fiber
	whole milk	skim milk	organic low-fat milk
	sweetened refined cereal	quick oats	steel-cut oats
	soy chicken	soy burgers	soybeans
	eggs	free-range/cage-free eggs	organic free-range eggs
	hamburger	lean ground beef	organic ground buffalo
	chicken nuggets	chicken	organic chicken
	fish sandwich	farm-raised salmon	wild Alaskan salmon
	white bread	whole-wheat bread	organic whole-grain sprouted bread
	partially hydrogenated peanut butter	natural peanut butter	organic peanut butter

How much protein is enough?

Protein has tremendous nutritional benefits when balanced correctly in your diet. Your goal should be to get 15 to 25 percent of your daily calories from high-quality protein sources, spread evenly throughout the day. The more physically active you are, the higher the amount of protein your body will need. Rarely does one need more than 25 percent of their daily calories from high-quality proteins. Another easy method is to take your body weight, cut it in half, and that number is the amount of protein in grams you need per day. So if you weigh 150 pounds, then you would need approximately 75 grams of protein per day. If you are eating more *whole foods* throughout the day, getting enough high-quality protein should not be a problem for most people.

Recommended protein consumption based on daily calorie intake		
Total calories	Grams of protein	Number of protein calories
1,200	45–75	180–300
1,500	56–94	225–375
1,800	68–113	270–450
2,000	75–125	300–500
2,500	94–156	375–625
3,000	113–188	450–750

What happens if I eat too much protein? Getting more than 25 percent of your daily calories from protein may cause the body to become too acidic (refer to Chapter 5 for more information on pH balance). When proteins are broken down, they must be neutralized by buffering elements, namely calcium, magnesium, and iodine, to offset the high acid levels in the body. If your protein intake is too high, these buffering elements may become depleted over time, which may lead to a decrease in bone mass, low thyroid, and digestion and absorption problems in the stomach and digestive tract. Eating too much protein also places stress on the liver and kidneys, which have to work harder to rid the body of the byproducts of excess protein metabolism. Remember, your first challenge is to look at the *quality* of proteins that you are using. Second, start to pay attention to the *quantity* of protein you are consuming.

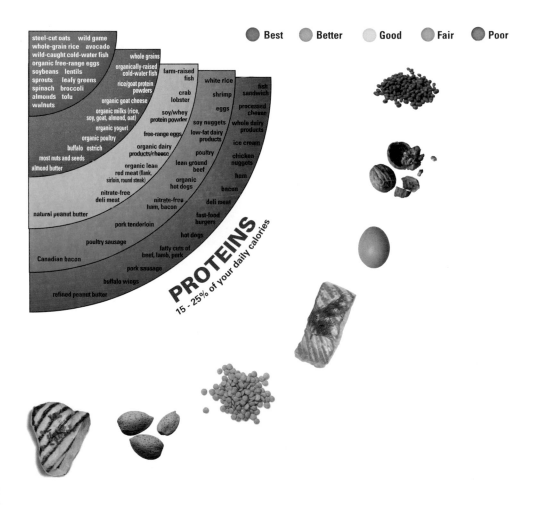

● Best ● Better ● Good ● Fair ● Poor

steel-cut oats   wild game
whole-grain rice   avocado
wild-caught cold-water fish
organic free-range eggs
soybeans   lentils
sprouts   leafy greens
spinach   broccoli
almonds   tofu
walnuts

whole grains
organically-raised cold-water fish
rice/goat protein powders
organic goat cheese
organic milks (rice, soy, goat, almond, oat)
organic yogurt
organic poultry
buffalo   ostrich
most nuts and seeds
almond butter
organic lean red meat (flank, sirloin, round steak)
nitrate-free deli meat
natural peanut butter
pork tenderloin
poultry sausage
Canadian bacon

farm-raised fish
crab
lobster
soy/whey protein powder
free-range eggs
organic dairy products/cheese
lean ground beef
organic hot dogs
nitrate-free ham, bacon
fast-food burgers
hot dogs
fatty cuts of beef, lamb, pork
pork sausage
buffalo wings
refined peanut butter

white rice
shrimp
eggs
soy nuggets
low-fat dairy products
poultry
ham
bacon
deli meat

fish sandwich
processed cheese
whole dairy products
ice cream
chicken nuggets

PROTEINS
15 - 25% of your daily calories

THE BOTTOM LINE

1. Proteins are important to the health and performance of the human body in many ways. Proteins are necessary for cell development, increased energy, to reduce cravings of refined carbohydrates, and improve brain power.
2. Proteins are broken down in the body into nitrogen-containing units called amino acids. There are twenty-two amino acids, nine essential and thirteen non-essential. The body cannot manufacture essential amino acids, so we must get them through the foods we eat.
3. Organic animal protein sources: If you choose to consume animal-based proteins, choose organic sources whenever possible.
4. Consume 15 to 25 percent of your daily calories from high-quality protein sources. An easy method to figure your daily protein intake is to take your body weight in pounds and cut it in half; this will give you grams of protein to consume per day.
5. Consider the quality, quantity, and frequency with which you eat protein.

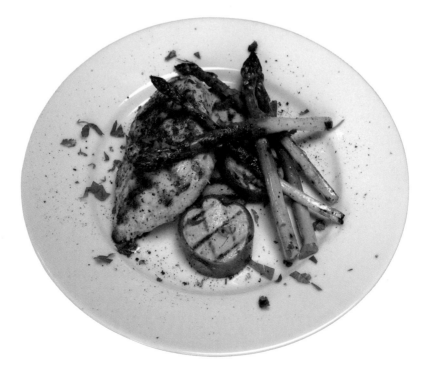

Chapter 12
HEAL YOUR BODY WITH FATS

We are a nation obsessed with a fear of fat. Sixty percent of Americans rank cutting fat as their number-one nutritional concern. You cannot walk through the grocery store aisles without seeing "fat free" plastered on every type of food imaginable. We have been led to believe that if a food has little or no fat, it must be okay to eat, and that foods containing fats should be avoided at all costs. This is flawed thinking. By the end of this chapter I want you to understand that eating healthy fats is one of the best things you can do to keep your body healthy, improve your energy, and perform at your best! *View healthy fats as your body's healing nutrients.*

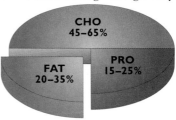

CHO 45–65%

PRO 15–25%

FAT 20–35%

In my On Target Living seminars, I spend a great deal of time explaining the benefits of eating quality fats and giving direction as to how much fat to consume daily. Nonetheless, it never fails that immediately following a discussion of quality fats, a participant will approach me to lament that extra-virgin olive oil or flaxseed oil—which I just recommended in the lecture—has fourteen grams of fat per tablespoon. I ask them if they had the same thought process when we were discussing carbohydrates (a half cup of oatmeal has twenty-seven grams of carbohydrate) or proteins (one chicken breast has twenty grams of protein). Until convinced about the importance of incorporating quality fats into the diet, many people just look at the labels, see the amount of fat, and wonder how I could possibly recommend that that much fat be added to their diets.

> Joy comes from using your potential.
>
> —Will Schultz

I see the same mindset with some of my personal training clients. A personal training client may seek my services with the goal of increasing energy, lowering cholesterol or blood pressure, controlling diabetes, decreasing inflammation, or simply losing weight. I spend considerable time explaining cellular health and the benefits of eating the right kinds of fats, cite research, share testimonials, and share my own experience with—and passion for—eating healthy fats. Clients with this information sometimes still reject the idea of adding any type of fat to their diet. Their response is "how could I ever use those extra calories?"

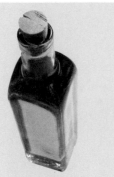

Extra-virgin olive oil

We have been led to believe that all fats are unhealthy and will cause us to gain weight and become fat—the old you-are-what-you-eat way of thinking. True, fats do contain over twice the calories per gram (nine calories) as carbohydrates and proteins (four calories). However, consuming healthy fats creates satiety, decreases the desire to overeat, balances hormones, decreases inflammation, and increases metabolic rate by fueling the power pack of our cells, the mitochondria!

One conclusion that can be drawn from recent medical research is that you don't have to give up fat to lose weight or enjoy better health. In fact, the opposite is true. Eating healthy fats is essential for better health, energy, and weight control.

So let me get this straight, by eating healthy fats I will improve my health, increase my energy, and control my weight? Absolutely! One of the primary goals of *On Target Living Nutrition* is to help you distinguish between healthy and unhealthy fats.

MEDICAL RESEARCH SUPPORTING HEALTHY FATS

The most definitive study showing the benefits of consuming healthy fats is the Seven Countries Study, a fifteen-year study that began in the 1950s. Pioneering nutrition researcher Ancel Keys and his colleagues looked at the eating patterns of sixteen populations in seven countries. Keys and his colleagues studied over 12,000 men from Greece, Italy, the Netherlands, Finland, Japan, Yugoslavia, and the United States. This study concluded that the people of the Greek island of Crete (eating a diet virtually unchanged since 4,000 B.C.) had the lowest death rates from cancer and heart disease. Crete had half the death rate from cancer and one-twentieth the death rate from heart disease of the United States. What is unique about the Cretan diet?

First, the overall fat intake is high—35 percent of their total calories comes from fat. Second, the types of fat consumed are much different than the types of fat consumed in the United States. The Cretan diet is low in trans-fatty acids (such as french fries, refined peanut butter, and margarine), refined saturated fats (such as whole dairy products, processed cheese, and fatty cuts of meat), and refined omega-6 fatty acids (such as corn, soy, and cottonseed oil), all unhealthy forms of fat. The Cretan diet is high in whole fruits, vegetables, leafy greens, raw nuts and seeds, extra-virgin olive oil, fish, and flaxseeds. The Cretan diet is loaded with simple unprocessed foods and a variety of healthy fats!

How did the U.S. compare? We continue to increase our intake of trans-fatty acids and saturated fats from processed snacks, fast food, and animal products. Americans are also consuming too many refined omega-6 fats and not enough omega-3 fats. As a result of our poor eating habits, we have seen a dramatic rise in:

- obesity
- Type 2 diabetes
- arthritis
- inflammation
- heart disease
- cancer
- depression
- dementia
- autoimmune diseases
- prescription medications

USA Obesity Rates
58 million overweight; 40 million obese; 3 million morbidly obese
Eight out of 10 over-25s overweight
78% of Americans not meeting basic activity level recommendations
25% completely sedentary
76% increase in Type II diabetes in adults 30–40 years old since 1990

SOURCE: Wellness International Network Ltd - web.winltd.com

WHERE HAVE WE GONE WRONG?

Since the early 1950s we have slowly decreased the quality of the fat we are consuming. The more refining or processing that goes into producing food, the more quality (healthy fat) is stripped away. We are a nation of convenience eaters. In return, we get unhealthy, refined, convenient food sources. Our entire food supply has been affected by our demand for convenience and packaged foods.

In his book *Fast Food Nation,* Eric Schlosser says, "Americans spend more on fast food than we spend on higher education, personal computers, new cars, movies, books, magazines, newspapers, videos, and recorded music combined."

Why do food manufacturers and the fast-food industry use poor-quality fat in packaging and preparing food?

1. **Money:** The two most consumed oils in the United States are refined soybean and corn oil. Refined soybean and corn oil are extremely abundant and inexpensive, and are used in thousands of food products to enhance taste. Next time you are at the grocery store, pick up a packaged food product and see if one of these evil twins is in the ingredient list. If they are, avoid these highly

refined omega-6 oils. Refined omega-6 fats are not healthy and lie in the orange area of the *Food Target*.

2. **Shelf life:** Manufacturers in the food industry understand that the longer a product can stay on the shelf without becoming stale or spoiling, the greater the profitability of that product. Manufacturers start with refined soybean or corn oil and take them through a process called *hydrogenation*. Hydrogenation is a process in which these refined oils are subjected to extreme heat and then a metal catalyst is added, turning these refined oils into *trans-fatty acids*. Trans-fats are extremely unhealthy and lie on the outer ring, the red area of the *Food Target*.

My first experience with hydrogenated food products started with one of my first jobs out of college. I took a job with a large snack-food company as a route sales-person. For almost seven years, eight hours a day, I lived in grocery stores, stocking shelves, putting up displays, and trying to acquire more shelf space to increase my sales. I observed shoppers in every shape and size and their buying practices. The experience and knowledge I gathered helped me understand the power of the food industry along with how many people truly do not understand what they are putting into their grocery carts and then into their precious bodies!

In my job I handled a variety of snack foods, including potato chips, tortilla chips, pretzels, and soft cookies. The chips and pretzels had a four- to-six-week shelf life before being returned as stale. The packaged soft cookies, on the other hand, had a shelf life of over thirty-six months—*three years!* In fact, after the soft cookies were returned to the warehouse as stale, they would be left out for the drivers to eat. Weeks would go by and the cookies were still soft! Can you imagine how hard your mom's homemade cookies would become if they were left out for a few weeks? Remember Ellie Mae Clampett from the television show the "Beverly Hillbillies"? She was such a lousy cook that even Jethro would not eat her cookies because he was afraid he would chip a tooth! This is what mom's cookies would be like if left out for weeks.

In my On Target Living seminars I try to make the point that once partially hydro-genated oils are used in a food product, the shelf life of that product is a long, long time! I have a jar of a well-known brand of refined peanut butter that I display for this very purpose. It has been in my garage for over thirteen years! If trans-fatty acids can pre-serve a bag of cookies for more than three years and a jar of refined peanut butter for more than thirteen years, think about the effect they have on your body once they are consumed.

These are just two examples of how unhealthy fats make their way into our cupboards and onto our dinner tables. In our society, we have to search for good fats while working overtime to avoid bad fats.

WHY IS EATING HEALTHY FATS SO ESSENTIAL TO OPTIMAL PERFORMANCE AND GOOD HEALTH?

The human body is made up of over 100 trillion cells. Each cell has a specific job to do and is in a constant state of change. On the most basic level, fats help form the membrane that surrounds each of our cells. The cell membrane controls the elements that enter and exit the cell. This is one of the major functions of the body that is threatened by eating unhealthy trans-fatty acids. Trans-fatty acids interfere with normal fat metabolism by crowding or pushing out essential fatty acids from cell membranes. This makes the cells less fluid and less permeable, and reduces the number and sensitivity of the insulin receptors.

When working with a client who has Type 2 diabetes or for that matter anyone who wants to become healthier, one of my first goals is to get their cells healthier, and this includes getting the cell membranes soft and permeable. A stiff and insensitive cell membrane is a major factor in Type 2 diabetes. When insulin approaches the cell and tries to open it up to allow nutrients to enter, it has a tougher time doing its job if trans-fatty acids have made the outer membrane of the cell rock solid like an M&M candy shell, hard on the outside, soft on the inside. Over time the cells become insulin-resistant and Type 2 diabetes may soon follow.

Replacing your unhealthy fats with healthy fats has amazing benefits. It is the first step to cellular health and having softer cell membranes that are more permeable and sensitive to insulin. Eating healthy fats also satisfies your hunger because healthy

Decreases	Improves
inflammation	the immune system
arthritis symptoms	brain development, cognitive skills, focus
cancer incidence	skin, hair, and nails
migraine headaches	absorption of vitamins
post-menopausal symptoms	weight loss
depression	"brown fat" for body temperature regulation
constipation	cardiovascular health
high blood pressure	hormonal balance
cholesterol	overall health and well-being
platelet aggregation	ADHD (attention deficit hyperactivity disorder)

fats cause the release of a hormone called cholecystokinin (CCK) from the stomach. CCK alerts the brain that you are satisfied. Without sufficient fat, you are more likely to overeat. Fats also slow down the digestion of carbohydrates and proteins so that there is a more sustained release of nutrients into the blood, resulting in a stable energy level. If you goal is to lose weight, lower your cholesterol, blood pressure, blood glucose, decrease inflammation, or just want to feel great, start replacing your unhealthy fats with healthy fats!

THE CATEGORIES OF FATS

Learning to distinguish between a healthy and an unhealthy fat is critical for good health and performance. There are four categories of fat to learn more about and understand:

1. Trans-fatty acids
2. Saturated fats
3. Monounsaturated fats (omega-9)
4. Polyunsaturated fats (omega-3 and omega-6 essential fatty acids)

Trans-fatty acids

These are the worst of the bad fats! Hydrogenating, or hardening, vegetable oils creates trans-fatty acids, also known as partially hydrogenated fats. As noted earlier, the food industry widely uses trans-fats because they are inexpensive, improve taste, and increase shelf life. Trans-fatty acids are difficult for the body to break down and impair the normal use of healthy fats by hardening the cell membrane. Trans-fatty acids raise LDL (bad) cholesterol and lower HDL (good) cholesterol, pushing both the bad and the good blood lipids in the wrong direction. Today, the average American consumes over 20 percent of his or her calories from trans-fatty acids. Studies show that *there is no acceptable level of trans-fats.*

Unless we are vigilant, it is easy to consume trans-fatty acids because they are hidden in almost all processed foods. Trans-fatty acids are found in margarine, shortening, doughnuts, french fries, pound cake, crackers, potato chips, packaged soft cookies, baked goods, microwave popcorn, non-dairy creamers, and refined peanut butter, to name a few.

In 2006, the Food and Drug Administration (FDA) required all food and beverages to list trans-fats on the label. So this is good news, right? Yes and no! I believe it will create more awareness on the detrimental affects that trans-fats have on the body, but the buyer needs to understand what to look for to avoid these unhealthy fats! Now, you may be thinking, I don't have to worry about trans-fats being in the food that I buy, I can just look at the label and it will tell me if the product has trans-fats or not. Not so fast. There is a little loophole that you need to know about the labeling of fats.

The FDA allows food manufacturers to label a product fat-free or trans-fat free if it contains less than half a gram of fat per serving. So what you are telling me is that a product may contain trans-fats, but the packaging can say it has zero trans-fats? Unfortunately, yes. The only way to truly know if a product contains trans-fats is to look at the ingredient list first. Any time the words *"hydrogenated"* or *"partially hydrogenated"* appear in the ingredient list, the product contains trans-fatty acids, regardless of whether the packaging says zero trans-fats.

Saturated fats

Can saturated fats be good for you? *It depends* on the quality of the saturated fat. Consumers have been told for years that saturated fats are unhealthy and are responsible for heart disease, cancer, obesity, and a host of degenerative diseases.

Do you really need saturated fats in your nutritional plan for better health and performance? The answer is yes! Healthy saturated fats give structural integrity to the cell. Just as you need a variety of fruits and vegetables to fill many of your nutrient requirements for vitamins, minerals, and antioxidants, the same is true when consuming healthy fats. Ideally, you want a variety of healthy fats in your eating plan to achieve the nutrient requirements your body needs.

How do you know if a saturated fat is healthy or unhealthy? Your best bet is to look for saturated fats in their most natural state (whole foods), just as you would with your selection of carbohydrates and proteins. Most saturated fats are solid at room temperature. Animal products such as meat, eggs, and dairy, as well as most seeds and nuts, all contain some saturated fat. The quality and amount of saturated fat in food depend on the quality of food the animals were eating and the environment in which they were raised. The best quality saturated fats come from animals raised under the most natural conditions (walking around grazing on grass, insects, and seeds). Most nuts and seeds are excellent sources of saturated fat, protein, and fiber.

One of the healthiest fats for the body just happens to also be a saturated fat. Can you guess what this wonderful fat could be? If you answered *organic extra-virgin coconut oil,* you were right! For years, consumers have been told that coconut oil is high in saturated fat and we

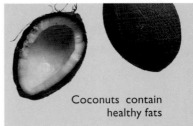

Coconuts contain healthy fats

should avoid it at all costs. I ask this question in my seminars, "Are saturated fats healthy or unhealthy?" The correct answer, *it depends!* It depends on the quality of the fat. Is the coconut found in a refined candy bar or out of a package that you sprinkle on a German chocolate cake? If you were on a tropical island and a coconut fell to the ground, do you think the coconut would be something healthy to eat or drink? The answer, yes! The fact is, coconuts have nourished humans for thousands of years! From skin problems to an upset stomach, coconut was the remedy of choice.

What makes organic extra-virgin coconut oil so special? It is rich in lauric, capric, and caprylic acids, which are loaded with antiviral and antifungal properties. Lauric acid is also present in breast milk.

Some of the wonderful health benefits of organic extra-virgin coconut oil include:
• aids digestive disorders (acid reflux, irritable bowel syndrome)
• weight loss
• promotes beautiful looking skin
• high in antioxidants
• improves thyroid function
• protects against heart disease

Organic extra-virgin coconut oil has a wonderful flavor and can be used as a butter replacement. It is also excellent for cooking and in recipes due to its stability under wide temperature ranges. I use it to spread on a cracker or a piece of toast, scramble eggs, in a smoothie drink, mixed in with my oatmeal, or just a spoonful in the evening. It makes me feel satisfied and curbs those evening food cravings that most of us struggle with. Oh, I almost forgot, I also give a little bit to my dog, Dolly. She loves the taste and it keeps her coat and tummy healthy!

Store your organic extra-virgin coconut oil in the cupboard at room temperature. It will melt easily if the temperature exceeds 76 degrees. Organic extra-virgin coconut oil can be found in most health-food stores. **Recommended serving: one to two tablespoons per day.**

Monounsaturated fats (omega-9 fats)

Monounsaturated fats (also know as omega-9 fats) play an important role in your balanced diet. Monounsaturated fats contain the fatty acid known as *oleic acid.*

Health benefits of monounsaturated fats

Monounsaturated fats protect the arteries from cholesterol buildup, reduce the risk of breast cancer, accentuate the effect of omega-3 fatty acids in the blood, and help in the formation and development of all cell membranes, which is important for cell, tissue, and organ health. One of the main reasons monounsaturated fats are so protective against heart disease is that they lower LDL (bad cholesterol) while they maintain or even raise HDL (good cholesterol) levels—the best of both worlds. *No other fat has this effect!*

Monounsaturated fats are preferred over polyunsaturated fats for cooking because they have a single double-bond between their carbon atoms, making them stable at high temperatures, not easily oxidized, and great-tasting. Anytime a recipe calls for oil, your best choices are monounsaturated fats and organic extra-virgin coconut oil.

Where do you find monounsaturated fats?

Monounsaturated fats are found in olives, extra-virgin olive oil, avocados, avocado oil, almonds, almond oil, almond butter, peanuts, natural peanut butter, macadamia nuts, macadamia oil, expeller-pressed canola oil, pistachio nuts, pecans, cashews, hazelnuts, and pine nuts. Monounsaturated fats are also found in high oleic expeller-pressed safflower and sunflower oils.

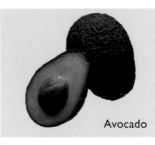

Avocado

What to look for when buying oils made from monounsaturated fats

The process of refining destroys many of the wonderful health benefits of oils and other products made from monounsaturated fats. Producers use refining techniques to improve profits without regard to the negative effect that refining has on the products and the consumer. Olive oil is a refined oil. Virgin olive oil is a better choice because it is less refined. Extra-virgin olive oil is even better. To be classified as extra-virgin olive oil, the oil must be from the first pressing, the highest quality, and extracted under strict adherence to specific guidelines. If olives are damaged or bruised, they begin to spoil. The oil that is pressed from these olives is of such poor quality that it must be refined, degummed, bleached, and deodorized, resulting in poor-quality olive oil. The processes used to mass-produce oils remove and strip many of the essential nutrients that provide critical health benefits. When selecting monounsaturated fats (oils, nuts, or seeds), choose only high-quality, unrefined

What 300 calories look like
• adding one large tablespoon of slivered almonds to your cereal for breakfast • adding one tablespoon of extra-virgin olive oil to your salad at lunch • adding one tablespoon of natural peanut butter or almond butter to a piece of whole-grain toast or apple as a snack *All of these together add up to 300 calories.*

sources whenever possible. Store all your monounsaturated fats at room temperature in a dark container or in the cupboard to maintain their high nutritional value.

How much monounsaturated fat should you eat?

Approximately 10 to 15 percent of your daily calories should come from monounsaturated fats. If you consume approximately 2,000 calories per day, roughly 200–300 calories (twenty to thirty grams, two to three tablespoons) should come from monounsaturated fats.

Polyunsaturated fatty acids—essential fatty acids

Polyunsaturated fats include essential fatty acids. This means we must obtain them from the foods we eat because our bodies don't produce them and they are *necessary* for proper function of our bodies. At the microscopic level, polyunsaturated fatty acids have two or more double-bonds in their carbon chains; the more double-bonds on the carbon chain, the more unsaturated the oil. Flaxseed and fish oil are the most unsaturated of all oils; this is one reason why you never want to heat or cook these oils. All polyunsaturated oils are liquid at room temperature and remain liquid when refrigerated.

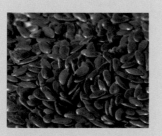
Flaxseed

In the past, we believed that any type of polyunsaturated fat was healthy, with little distinction between types of polyunsaturated fatty acids. We now understand that polyunsaturated fats fall into two distinct groups: *omega-3* and *omega-6 essential fatty acids,* each aiding specific functions in the body. The type and refinement or processing is important with regard to the quality and benefit of these fats.

With all the refinement of our foods today, 92 percent of U.S. adults are deficient in these essential fatty acids. When working with clients one-on-one, I have them turn in a two- or three-day food log to get a better understanding of how they fuel their bodies. I rarely see essential fatty acids in their nutritional plan. Most don't know what an essential fatty acid is, and, most importantly, where to find them. In the past, our entire food chain—greens, eggs, meat, nuts, seeds, and fish—contained these wonderful essential fatty acids. We all were eating more whole foods that delivered these wonderful essential fatty acids to our bodies. Unfortunately this is not the case today; we have to search for these fats.

Omega-3 essential fatty acids

Omega-3 fats are the superstars of the healthy fats and make the body strong and healthy. The primary fatty acid in the omega-3 family is *alpha-linolenic acid* (LNA). LNA is found in green leafy vegetables, flax meal, flaxseed oil, walnuts, brazil nuts, pumpkin seeds, and pumpkin seed oil. Flax meal and flaxseed oil are the richest sources of LNA.

There are three levels of omega-3 breakdowns, or conversions, in the body. LNA converts to one of two other types of fatty acids, depending upon its breakdown pathway. LNA is converted into eicosapentaenoic acid (EPA) and then into docosahexaenoic acid (DHA). Scientists became aware of the wonderful health benefits of EPA and DHA when Danish physicians observed that Greenland Eskimos had exceptionally low incidences of heart disease and arthritis, despite the fact that they consumed a high-fat diet! The type of fat the Greenland Eskimos were consuming was high in EPA and DHA, found in cold-water fish such as salmon, trout, tuna, mackerel, and herring, and in cod liver and fish oils.

People attending my On Target Living seminars often ask, "If I eat omega-3 fats, such as flax meal or flaxseed oil, which is high in LNA, do I also need to consume wild cold-water fish and cod liver or fish oils?" Ideally, yes! The conversion from LNA to EPA and then into DHA is not efficient in most adults and especially in seniors and children. I recommend one serving of flax and fish oil on a daily basis to fill all of your omega-3 essential fatty acid needs. If you are just trying to make a few changes to begin with, don't worry about doing everything on day one! Get comfortable with your new changes and then down the road you may want to do both (flax and fish oils).

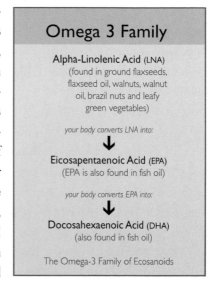

Omega 3 Family

Alpha-Linolenic Acid (LNA)
(found in ground flaxseeds, flaxseed oil, walnuts, walnut oil, brazil nuts and leafy green vegetables)

your body converts LNA into:
↓

Eicosapentaenoic Acid (EPA)
(EPA is also found in fish oil)

your body converts EPA into:
↓

Docosahexaenoic Acid (DHA)
(also found in fish oil)

The Omega-3 Family of Ecosanoids

Benefits of consuming omega-3 fats

Weight loss with omega-3 fats. Many people are surprised to hear that consuming fats, especially the right types of fats, can actually help you to lose weight! They are concerned that if they add more calories to their own food plan, weight gain will most certainly follow. I recently had a young woman at one of my seminars ask "the question":

"So let me get this straight, you are recommending to this entire audience to consume approximately 400 to 800 calories per day of good fats?" Everyone is waiting for the answer because many were thinking the same thing. My answer was a most definite "yes!" *First,* going back to the cell, remember the cell membrane and the mitochondria? When you start eating the healthy fats, the cell membrane becomes healthier and the mitochondria get more metabolically active. *Second,* good fats make you feel satisfied and help control appetite, food cravings, and most importantly your blood glucose level. *Third,* with greater energy you want to move your body more.

Hormonal balance with omega-3 fats. Polyunsaturated fatty acids are important for creating hormonal balance in the body. Both the omega-3 and omega-6 fats work by forming short-lived, hormone-like substances called prostaglandins. Prostaglandins regulate metabolic processes throughout the body at the cellular level. They control cellular communication and are essential in regulating the immune, reproductive, central nervous, and cardiovascular systems.

Healthy heart with omega-3 fats. Prostaglandins formed from omega-3 fats aid in the cardiovascular system by reducing constriction of blood vessels and decreasing the stickiness of the blood, making it less likely to clot. Eating too much unhealthy (trans-fatty acids, refined saturated, and omega-6) fats and not eating enough of the omega-3 fats will likely create a prostaglandin imbalance. Omega-3 fats help to maintain elasticity of artery walls, prevent blood clotting, reduce blood pressure, and stabilize heart rhythm.

High cholesterol is a growing concern in the United States and throughout the world. Cholesterol-lowering medications are as common as aspirin. Is there a better way? What are MY options? Start by getting your cells healthy! Get the trans-fats out of your diet, drink more water, eat more whole foods, add one or two tablespoons of flax meal to your cereal or glass of juice, add one or two teaspoons of fish oil, and work closely with your physician.

Over the past decade, I have received hundreds of emails, letters, and phone calls, and I even had one person waiting to greet me before one of my seminars, all wanting to share their personal stories on the dramatic improvements to their health and cholesterol levels! Yes, you do have options!

Diabetics' need for omega-3 fats. Anytime I have an opportunity to work with someone who has diabetes, I get very excited about sharing with them the power of eating the "healthy fats," whether they have Type 1 diabetes (their body is no longer producing insulin) or Type 2 diabetes (their body is still producing insulin, but the cells are not receptive to the insulin that is produced). Again, back to the cell! Step number one: get the cell membrane soft and receptive to insulin. As the cell membrane becomes softer and more sensitive, the demand for insulin decreases. Regular exercise, drinking water, eating whole foods, and consuming healthy fats go a long way in making the cell membrane more sensitive. It sounds pretty simple: exchange the unhealthy fats with the healthy fats, especially the omega-3 fats. Remember, your body is always trying to heal itself! If you have Type 1 or Type 2 diabetes, work with your healthcare professional and start getting healthy fats into your nutritional plan.

TAKE IT FROM ME...

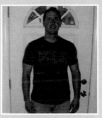

My epiphany came one morning when I stepped on the scale and finally realized I had reached a fork in the road. I was twenty-five years old, newly married, and convinced I was walking a path that led to a lifestyle I didn't want or was willing to continue. Coming from a family history with heart problems, diabetes, and high blood pressure, I knew what things I had to look forward to if I didn't start to make some changes! As a former college football player I knew the benefits of a healthy lifestyle and wanted to get my body back in the shape I was once in. The problem was I just didn't know how I was going to do it.

**Regie Rieder, age 25,
Lansing, Michigan**

When I learned about Chris Johnson and his On Target Living Program I could feel his sincerity and strong belief in what he was teaching and knew he was the person who would change my life. After one of his seminars and a few days with his book, I began to realize the extreme level of importance proper nutrition and exercise holds in our life not only physically, but mentally and emotionally as well. Since beginning his program six months ago I have lost thirty-five pounds and I still am amazed at the amount of energy I have every day to do the things in my life that I love. I feel better physically now at the age of twenty-five than I did at eighteen and cannot wait to continue reaching the lofty goals Chris Johnson's program has helped me believe I can obtain. I encourage anyone wanting to make some healthy changes in their life no matter large or small, to embrace On Target Living, believe in what it teaches, and allow it to change your life forever!

Reduced inflammation with omega-3 fats. We all know what inflammation is! You get stung by a bee and your arm swells up. Or you sprain your ankle, and it swells up. But what about the chronic inflammation that affects millions of people on a daily basis? Have you ever wondered why some people have more inflammation than others? Do you ever feel like you have been in a train wreck when you get out of bed in the morning? Would you like to have fewer aches and pains? I think most people don't link inflammation to their diets. Could it be connected to what we are eating or not eating? Most people don't realize that *omega-3 fats have natural anti-inflammatory* *benefits!* Eating and drinking the right foods and beverages are powerful ways to decrease inflammation. Instead of purchasing an over-the-counter or prescription anti-inflammatory, begin using omega-3 fats as your anti-inflammatory of choice!

Your brain needs DHA. The omega-3 fat docosahexaenoic (DHA) is the building block of human brain tissue and is abundant in the grey matter of the brain and the retina of the eye. Low levels of DHA have recently been associated with depression, memory loss, dementia, and visual problems. DHA is particularly important for fetal and infant development. The DHA content of an infant's brain triples during the first three months of life! Optimal levels of DHA are, therefore, crucial for pregnant and lactating mothers. Unfortunately, the average DHA content in breast milk in the U.S. is the lowest in the world, most likely due to our failure to consume enough omega-3 fats.

Dr. Barbara Levine, professor of nutrition in medicine at Cornell University, sounds the alarm concerning the inadequate intake of DHA by most Americans. Dr. Levine believes that common health problems in the U.S., such as postpartum depression, attention deficit hyperactivity disorder (ADHD), and low IQ, are linked to low DHA intake. Dr. Levine also points out that low DHA levels have been linked to low serotonin levels. Serotonin is the "feel-good" neurotransmitter that is boosted by consuming omega-3 fats containing DHA. Moms, get busy consuming the proper omega-3 fats to keep you and baby or babies happy and healthy!

Personally, I have been consuming flax and fish oil for years. I sometimes wonder where I would be without my omega-3 fats. Sometimes I have to laugh at myself when I can't remember where I parked my car, or how to spell the word "the," or am feeling a little blue. It is just like the bald guy who is trying to keep his hair by using hair-growth lotion and you ask, does that stuff really work? He responds by stating, "I don't really know, but I can't afford to stop using it!" Omega-3 fats are worth making the effort to incorporate them into your diet every day. Like I ask my clients, "Do you brush your teeth every day?" They all say the same thing, "Of course, I do." Then create a similar ritual for taking your omega-3 fats. They are truly magical!

Where do you find omega-3 fats?

It is a challenge to get enough omega-3 fats unless you know where to look. I tell my clients, "You must search for omega-3 fats." Why is that? Omega-3 fats are extremely unstable and spoil quickly. Most products that are sitting in the grocery store do not contain omega-3 fats. There are, however, excellent sources of omega-3 fats available.

Flaxseeds. Flaxseeds have been around for thousands of years, making them one of mankind's earliest food supplies. In the eighth century, Charlemagne considered flax so essential for health that he passed laws requiring its use.

Flaxseeds are tiny, hard seeds, either gold or brown, that are loaded with omega-3 fatty acids. The seeds themselves *are not digestible,* so to reap the wonderful health benefits of the omega-3 fatty acids, the seeds must be ground into flax meal or pressed into flaxseed oil. Flaxseeds are inexpensive and are an excellent dietary source of fiber. Flaxseeds contain lignans, which have antiviral, antifungal, antibacterial, and anticancer properties. Lignans are found in the

> Wherever flaxseeds become a regular food item among the people, there will be better health.
>
> —Mahatma Gandhi

seed coat and only a small amount of lignans end up in the oil. If you want the benefits of lignans, use fresh ground seeds (flax meal). Whole flaxseeds may be used on salads or cereals or in baking. Whole flaxseeds are high in fiber and help curb appetite, but you lose some of the nutritional benefits, as stomach acid will not break down the whole seed.

Flax meal. Flax meal is ground flaxseeds. Flax meal is sold in health food stores, but I recommend that you purchase whole flaxseeds and grind your own to ensure freshness and maximum nutritional value. Buy a cheap coffee grinder specifically to grind your flaxseeds. I use the golden flaxseeds, which are a little sweeter. Once a week, I grind two cups of flaxseeds and place them in a container and store it in the refrigerator. This takes only couple of minutes and lasts the entire week. The flax meal is fresh and costs only pennies per day! Flax meal may be added to a variety of foods or beverages such as a glass of juice, smoothie, cereal, salads, or yogurt and adds a nutty flavor. **The recommended daily serving of flax meal is one to two tablespoons per hundred pounds of bodyweight.**

Flaxseed oil. An overwhelming amount of research has been done on the benefits of flax meal and flaxseed oil. Ground flax meal and flaxseed oil are the richest sources of the omega-3 fatty acids (LNA). You can find flaxseed oil in the refrigerated section of your local health or natural foods store. Flaxseed oil *must be refrigerated* and you should pay close attention to the date on the container—it has a shelf life of only a few months! *Do not heat or cook with flaxseed oil,* as heat destroys the omega-3 fats. I like the convenience and taste of the flaxseed oil, but it is more expensive and does not have the fiber benefits of the flax meal. Flaxseed oil may be added to cereal, smoothies, yogurt, or cottage cheese, or drizzled on a salad—be creative with it. When traveling, you may substitute flaxseed oil capsules for flaxseed oil, but it is expensive and may require a dose of twelve capsules, depending on your weight. **The recommended daily serving of flaxseed oil is one tablespoon (6,200 milligrams or six grams) per hundred pounds of body weight.** Just a reminder, pick the flax meal or the flaxseed oil each day, mix it up. On the days that I take a smoothie to work I use the flax meal in my smoothie. If I am not having a smoothie, I will use the flaxseed oil in my oatmeal. Experiment with flax and enjoy all the wonderful benefits it brings to you!

Forms	Health benefits	Use	Storage
Flaxseeds	Great source of dietary fiber and helps to curb appetite	Sprinkle one to two tablespoons on cereal, salads, or yogurt or use for baking	Store at room temperature for up to one year
Flax meal	Provides the most breast cancer–fighting lignans of any food (if they're not ground, the seeds can't provide the lignans)	Sprinkle one to two tablespoons on cereal or salads, in smoothies, or add to your favorite muffin recipe	Store in airtight container in refrigerator. May also be frozen.
Flaxseed oil	Best source of alpha-linolenic acid, which fights heart disease, breast cancer, and depression	Add to cereals or salads, drizzle over bread, or add to favorite smoothies, but don't use for cooking (heat breaks it down)	Buy refrigerated oil, and store in the refrigerator for six to eight weeks. Discard if it smells "fishy" or "painty."

There are many other sources of omega-3 fatty acids (LNA) such as walnuts, butternuts, brazil nuts, filberts, walnut oil, pumpkin seeds, pumpkin seed oil, hemp oil, and soybeans. Many of these nuts and oils contain omega-3, omega-6, and omega-9 fats. Leafy greens also contain small amounts of LNA.

Wonderful fish oils. As stated earlier, eicosapentaenoic (EPA) and docosahexaenoic (DHA) acids can be manufactured in small amounts by healthy cells from alpha-linolenic acid (LNA), which is found in great quantities in flax meal and flaxseed oil. However, the conversion from LNA to EPA and DHA is small and can be impaired by degenerative conditions such as diabetes. To directly get EPA and DHA into your body, take advantage of the wonderful benefits of fish oil. The richest sources of EPA and DHA are anchovies, herring, mackerel, oysters (farmed), wild salmon

(Alaska), salmon (canned pink/sockeye), and sardines. Unfortunately, much of the fish we consume in the United States today is not what it used to be years ago. Most of the salmon we buy today is farm-raised, and many other sources of fish contain levels of mercury, PCBs, and pesticides. Personally, I eat fresh fish on a regular basis. I love the taste of wild Alaskan salmon, but it is expensive. I also buy canned wild Alaskan salmon or canned light tuna and use on my salad two or three times a week.

To get the health benefits that fish oils provide I recommend to almost all my clients to take fish oil or cod liver oil daily. Did I read this right, cod liver oil? Hold on, this is not the nasty-tasting cod liver oil many of us had to take as a kid or when we got into trouble. Buy the fish oil and cod liver oil at your local health food store and ask the clerk for a recommendation. Not all fish oils are made with the same specifications. Also, I would recommend you buy the flavored cod liver oil. It comes in lemon and other fruit flavors. My mom is my taste tester, and she puts lemon-flavored cod liver oil in her yogurt. I put two teaspoons of cod liver oil in my cold oatmeal daily. My kids take it straight and wash it down with juice. Whatever way you want to use it is okay, just do it! As for the fish oils, one teaspoon contains approximately 400 mg of EPA and 550 mg of DHA. **Recommended daily serving size of fish or cod liver oil is one to three teaspoons.**

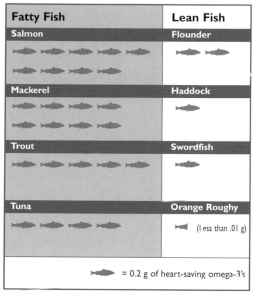

Fatty Fish	Lean Fish
Salmon	Flounder
Mackerel	Haddock
Trout	Swordfish
Tuna	Orange Roughy (Less than .01 g)

= 0.2 g of heart-saving omega-3's

How much omega-3 fats should you eat?

The question is, do you need both flax and fish oils to reach your daily requirements for omega-3 fatty acids? Ideally, the answer is yes. If you are just starting to use the flax, and that has been a major change for you, then leave it at

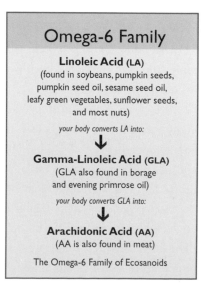

Omega-6 Family

Linoleic Acid (LA)
(found in soybeans, pumpkin seeds, pumpkin seed oil, sesame seed oil, leafy green vegetables, sunflower seeds, and most nuts)

your body converts LA into:

↓

Gamma-Linoleic Acid (GLA)
(GLA also found in borage and evening primrose oil)

your body converts GLA into:

↓

Arachidonic Acid (AA)
(AA is also found in meat)

The Omega-6 Family of Ecosanoids

that. As your habits begin to change you may want to add the fish or cod liver oil to your plan.

Flax and fish oils are truly magical in the health benefits they bring to the body. Whether you have high cholesterol, diabetes, inflammation, depression, or are struggling with your weight, these wonderful omega-3 fats can make a difference.

Omega-6 essential fatty acids

The second type of polyunsaturated fat comprises omega-6 fatty acids. The primary fatty acid in the omega-6 family is *linoleic acid* (LA). Vegetable oils such as corn, soybean, cottonseed, safflower, sunflower, pumpkin seed, and sesame seed all contain linoleic acid. It is also found in many nuts, seeds, and leafy greens. Animal sources of omega-6 fatty acids include lean meats, organ meats, and breast milk.

As in the omega-3 fatty acid family, which converts LNA to EPA and DHA, the primary omega-6 fatty acid converts into two fatty acids, gamma-linolenic acid (GLA) and arachidonic acid (AA).

Like the omega-3 family, the omega-6 family contains essential fatty acids. The body cannot produce these essential fatty acids, so they must come from the food we eat.

Health benefits of omega-6 essential fatty acids

As with omega-3 fats, omega-6 fats are essential for optimal health. Omega-6 fats are necessary for production of prostaglandins, the short-lived, hormone-like substances that regulate most of the body's life-sustaining systems. The body produces prostaglandins from the essential fatty acids we consume each day.

How is your brown fat working?

Our bodies have two types of fat cells, white fat and brown fat. White fat is the fat under the skin that insulates the body and is used for energy. This is the fat most of us are trying to lose.

Brown fat is the substance surrounding the organs and differs from white fat in many ways. Brown fat acts as a thermostat and helps the body acclimate to hot and cold temperatures. It aids in weight loss by helping the body convert calories into heat via thermogenesis. Brown fat helps burn 25 percent of all fat calories. In this regard, brown fat is an important element in metabolism.

As we age, brown fat begins to lose its burning capability. Think about the differences between senior citizens, who are often sensitive to the cold and gain weight in their late years, and youngsters, who are height-weight proportionate and tolerate cold temperatures easily. Most young children have metabolically active brown fat. I remember going to my grandparents' home as a kid and the heat would be cranked way up. It felt like a sauna. I never understood why they always felt cold; this was especially true in the winter months. As kids, we all remember being told put on our coats so we would not catch a cold! I remember putting my coat on to please my mom, but as soon as I was out of her sight, off came the coat!

How do you increase your brown fat? *Gamma-linolenic acid* (GLA), like its twin from the omega-3 family (EPA and DHA), helps fight heart disease, cancer, diabetes, inflammation, and arthritis, and also promotes weight loss. GLA in your daily diet is the raw material needed by the prostaglandins to stimulate brown fat. Dietary deficiencies and disease may block or slow the conversion of LA into GLA. This is one reason it may be necessary to find a direct source that contains GLA. *The highest source of GLA is evening primrose oil.*

Where do you find omega-6 fatty acids?

Just as you must search for omega-3 fatty acids, you must also search for high-quality, unrefined omega-6 fatty acids. The best sources of unrefined omega-6 fatty acids are soybeans, pumpkin seeds, pumpkin seed oil, sunflower seeds, sunflower seed oil, sesame seeds, sesame seed oil, evening primrose oil, black currant oil, flax meal, flaxseed oil, and leafy greens. Most raw nuts also contain omega-6 fatty acids. To get adequate amounts of GLA into your diet, use unrefined evening primrose or black currant oil. You must protect omega-6 fatty acids, just like omega-3 fatty acids, by buying them fresh and storing them safely in the refrigerator or freezer. *Do not heat or cook with omega-3 or omega-6 fats.* Heat destroys the benefits of these oils. Use only saturated fats such as extra-virgin coconut oil and most monounsaturated fats for cooking.

Arachidonic acid overload

Unlike omega-3 fatty acids, which are universally healthy fats, there are great differences in the quality and health benefits of omega-6 fats. Arachidonic acid (AA) is the end-product of omega-6 fatty acid conversions (LA-GLA-AA). The body needs some arachidonic acid to function optimally, but too much can promote poor health. Refined oils, such as corn or soybean oil, along with meat, especially red meat, can lead to arachidonic overload. To correct this, try to consume more unrefined oils and limit your consumption of red meat, refined oils, and processed foods. *Do not use refined omega-6 oils such as corn, soybean, cottonseed, and safflower oils!*

Omega-3 fats also help by blocking out the conversion to arachidonic acid, keeping your essential fats in balance.

How much omega-6 fat should you eat?

Make an effort to get one or two servings (one or two tablespoons) of unrefined, high-quality omega-6 fats in your diet each day. Include unrefined oils, raw nuts, seeds, or leafy greens in your daily diet.

Omega-3 and omega-6 fats in balance

Your body functions best when your diet contains a balanced ratio of omega-3 and omega-6 fatty acids. The World Health Organization recommends a two-to-one ratio of essential fatty acids: two parts omega-6 fats to one part omega-3 fat. In the United States, we generally eat an unbalanced ratio of omega-3 and omega-6 fatty acids. We have a sixteen-to-one (or greater) omega-6 to omega-3 ratio. Ouch!

This imbalance may lead to heart disease, diabetes, cancer, obesity, arthritis, inflammation, Alzheimer's disease, and a host of other autoimmune diseases. A large percentage of the American population over the age of forty-five is regularly taking self-prescribed, over-the-counter anti-inflammatory drugs like aspirin and ibuprofen.

Sample day of fats

BEGINNING:
1. **Cut the trans-fatty acids out of your diet.** Improve the quality of your peanut butter, crackers, chips, pizza—anything that may contain trans-fats.
2. **Add one or two tablespoons of flax meal or flaxseed oil.** You can consume this in your cereal, on a salad, in a smoothie drink, or with a glass of juice.

MODERATE:
1. **Add one or two tablespoons of raw nuts or seeds.** Add a few almonds, walnuts, pine nuts, and sesame, pumpkin, or sunflower seeds to your cereal or your favorite salad, or eat a handful as a snack.
2. **Add one or two tablespoons of extra-virgin olive oil or an avocado.** Add a tablespoon of extra-virgin olive oil or a slice of avocado to your favorite salad.
3. **Add one or two tablespoons of flax meal or flaxseed oil.** Put this in your cereal, on a salad, in a cup of yogurt or cottage cheese, in a smoothie drink, or with a glass of juice.

ADVANCED:
1. **Add one or two tablespoons of raw nuts or seeds.** As above.
2. **Add one tablespoon of organic extra-virgin coconut oil.** Organic extra-virgin coconut oil is excellent for cooking at high temperatures, and tastes great on a cracker or a piece of toast or melted over popcorn.
3. **Add one or two tablespoons of extra-virgin olive oil or avocado.** As above.
4. **Add one or two tablespoons of flax meal or flaxseed oil.** As above.
5. **Add one to three teaspoons of cod liver oil or fish oil.** Flavored cod liver oil or fish oil can be used on your cereal (this is how I take it), on a salad, in a smoothie, in a cup of cottage cheese or yogurt, or taken straight with a glass of juice.
6. **Add one or two teaspoons of evening primrose oil.** You can take this in capsule or liquid form and in the same manner as flax or fish oil.

These anti-inflammatory drugs may address the symptoms but not the underlying causes, which may be due to an imbalance in the consumption of omega-3 and omega-6 fats. Consequently, many modern-day health problems can be relieved by bringing these fatty acids into balance.

Since the 1960s, the U.S. consumption of omega-6 oils has doubled. One of the reasons the U.S. population is overeating omega-6 fats is that they are in almost every refined or processed food we consume. With technological improvements in oil extraction over the last sixty years, oil manufacturers can use inexpensive raw materials, such as corn and soybeans, and deliver a tremendous amount of this low-grade oil that is then used in thousands of products delivered to our grocery stores and fast-food restaurants. Next time you are in the grocery store, don't be shocked if you see these refined oils everywhere.

IMPROVING THE QUALITY OF FAT IN YOUR DIET

Don't become overwhelmed by trying to balance out your omega-3 and omega-6 fats. Start by removing all the *refined* oils such as corn, soy, cottonseed, safflower, and canola oils from your cupboard or refrigerator. Replace all your old, refined cooking oils with high-quality saturated and monounsaturated oils. Then move to high-quality omega-3 and omega-6 fats such as flax meal, flaxseed oil, fish oils, evening primrose oil, most nuts and seeds, and leafy greens. Most high-quality omega-3 fats also contain omega-6 fats.

I have outlined a sample day of consuming healthy fats. *Your goal is to improve the quality along with getting a greater variety of healthy fats in your diet.* Experiment with how you are taking these healthy fats.

Consuming healthy fats is magical in developing a healthy body. Develop consistent patterns in consuming your healthy fats.

Recommended fat consumption based on daily calorie intake		
Total calories	Grams of fat	Number of fat calories
1,200	27–47	240–420
1,500	33–58	300–525
1,800	40–70	360–630
2,000	44–78	400–700
2,500	56–97	500–875
3,000	67–117	600–1,050

THE BOTTOM LINE

1. Healthy fats are your body's healing nutrient.
2. Healthy fats make you feel satisfied, improve your energy, and create hormonal balance.
3. Your goal is to eat a variety of high-quality saturated, monounsaturated (omega-9), omega-3, and omega-6 fats on a daily basis.
4. Avoid trans-fats, refined saturated fats, and refined omega-6 fats.
5. Your goal is to consume four to eight tablespoons of healthy fats each day.

There is no other nutrient available that can heal the body and keep it healthy from infancy to old age like healthy fats.

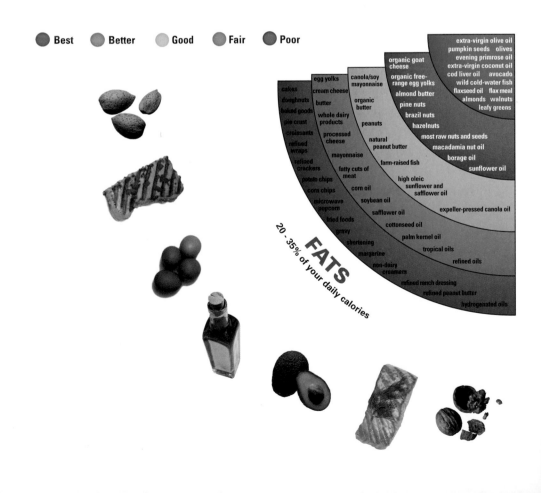

FAT SUMMARY GUIDE

Type	Trans-Fats	Saturated	Mono-unsaturated (Omega-9)	Poly-unsaturated (Omega-3)	Poly-unsaturated (Omega-6)
Source/quality	POOR: margarine, shortening, refined peanut butter, doughnuts, croissants, pie crust, cakes, non-dairy creamer, microwave popcorn, candy bars, refined snacks, baked goods, partially hydrogenated food products	BEST: organic extra-virgin coconut oil or raw coconut BETTER: wild game, organic cage-free egg yolks, most raw nuts and seeds, feta/goat cheese GOOD: organic butter, canola or soy mayonnaise FAIR: egg yolks, butter, dairy products POOR: refined tropical oils, fractionated oils, processed meat and cheese	BEST: organic extra-virgin olive oil, olives, avocados, almonds BETTER: almond butter, almond oils, pecans, cashews, pistachio nuts, macadamia nuts and oil, brazil nuts, pine nuts, most raw nuts and seeds GOOD: natural peanut butter, expeller-pressed canola oil, high oleic safflower and sunflower oils	BEST: cod liver oil, wild cold-water fish, flax meal, flaxseed oil, walnuts, leafy greens BETTER: most raw nuts and seeds	BEST: soybeans, hemp, sesame seeds, pumpkin seeds, evening primrose oil BETTER: most raw nuts and seeds, borage oil, sunflower oil POOR: refined corn oil, soybean oil, cottonseed oil, refined oils
Health benefits	detrimental to your health	wonderful health benefits when using unrefined sources	wonderful health benefits when using unrefined sources	wonderful health benefits when using unrefined sources	wonderful health benefits when using unrefined sources
Uses	used in refined foods to enhance taste and increase shelf life	great for cooking, baking, and spreads	great for cooking, baking, salads, and spreads	• DO NOT heat these fats • use in salads, cereal, smoothies • store in refrigerator	• DO NOT heat these fats • use in salads, cereal, smoothies • store in refrigerator
Serving size	avoid these harmful, unhealthy fats	½ to 1 tablespoon/day	2 to 3 tablespoons/day	1 to 2 tablespoons/day	1 to 2 tablespoons/day

The Chinese Bamboo

In the Far East the people plant a tree called the Chinese bamboo. During the first four years they water and fertilize the plant with seemingly little or no results. Then in the fifth year they again apply water and fertilizer—and in five weeks' time the tree grows ninety feet in height!

The obvious question is: did the Chinese bamboo tree grow ninety feet in five weeks, or did it grow ninety feet in five years? The answer is, it grew ninety feet in five years. Because if at any time during those five years the people had stopped watering and fertilizing the tree, it would have died.

Many times our dreams and plans appear not to be succeeding. We are tempted to give up and quit trying. Instead we need to continue to water and fertilize those dreams and plans.

Five Weeks

Year One   Year Two   Year Three   Year Four   Year Five

Chapter 13
CHECK YOUR FLUIDS

Over the last forty years, the types and quantities of beverages we consume have changed as dramatically as the foods we eat.

SODA POP

Soda pop is the number-one beverage in the United States. Number one! The average American drinks over seventy gallons of soda pop per year. I am doing the math on this, **300 million people × 70 gallons = 3 billion gallons of soda pop per year consumed in the United States.** Ouch! This number continues to grow, especially among our children and teenagers.

In my work and travels, the first beverage option I am usually given is soda pop. I was at a gas station not too long ago and this guy comes in to get a refill of his forty-four-ounce soda pop. Forty-four ounces! I try not to be the food police, but how can you not notice a forty-four-ounce cup? You have to be pretty strong just to hold onto that monster!

When I travel, one the first things I like to do is go out and get a few food and drink items while I am staying at my hotel. In many hotel rooms you have a prestocked refrigerator full of

> Those who bring the sunshine to the lives of others cannot keep it from themselves.
>
> —James Barrie

junk. Most hotel rooms do not have separate refrigerators. Not long ago I opened the refrigerated snack bar to make room for the food and drink items I had just purchased. I did a quick inventory of the choices and I was shocked. I knew there were many unhealthy choices, but I never would have believed the volume. There were twenty-nine drink and food items to choose from: four different choices of soda pop and beer, three alcoholic beverages, cookies, chips, candy bars, you name it, if it was loaded with trans-fats, high-fructose corn syrup, sugar, caffeine, or alcohol, it was in there! Until consumers demand higher-quality food and beverage choices, this trend will continue.

The most negative implication of the upward trend in soda pop consumption is the corresponding increase in sugar, artificial sweeteners, and phosphoric acid. On average, each American consumes over 185 pounds of sugar and over 25 pounds of artificial sweeteners per year! Too much sugar, artificial sweeteners, and phosphoric acid can lead to myriad health problems, such as obesity, Type 2 diabetes, inflammation, headaches, constipation, acid reflux, poor bone health, and low energy. If you are feeling tired and stressed, maybe it's time to cut back or slowly wean yourself off your soda pop altogether.

When my personal training clients wish to wean themselves off soda pop, I have them switch over to mineral water with a shot of fruit juice. My favorite is organic cherry or pomegranate juice. They enjoy the naturally occurring carbonation from the mineral water and a little sweetness from the fruit juice. Mineral water is alkaline, curbs your appetite, and is refreshing. If you have an occasional soda pop, not to worry, but if you find yourself drinking multiple servings per day and don't like how you feel, then maybe it's time to make some changes.

COFFEE

Drink coffee in moderation, one or two cups a day.

Americans just love their coffee. Coffee shops are virtually everywhere, and ordering a cup of coffee now has a language all its own. People enjoy the taste, aroma, warmth, and quick pick-me-up that coffee provides. For many, drinking a cup of coffee is a big part of their morning ritual. My recommendation is to drink coffee in moderation, one or two cups a day, and improve the quality of your coffee. Choosing organic coffee, whether regular or decaffeinated, is your best choice. Coffee, by nature, is acidic. Higher-quality, organic coffee is less acidic.

If you use some form of creamer in your coffee, avoid partially hydrogenated oils. Many creamers contain these unhealthy trans-fats. There are many healthy creamers to choose from that taste great and are good for you.

TEA

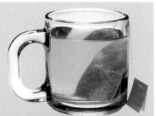

Enjoy the wonderful benefits tea may bring!

Tea is the most widely consumed beverage in the world, second only to water. For years, followers of alternative medicine have touted the health benefits of drinking tea. There are many different types of tea to choose from, such as white tea, oolong tea, black tea, and green tea. Green tea has attracted more and more followers as the word spreads about its health and medicinal benefits. Green tea is high in catechins, antioxidants that block the action of harmful free radicals. A free radical is an atom or group of atoms that contains one or more unpaired electrons. Free radicals are like thieves and will steal electrons from other paired electrons. Free radicals are hungry little buggers and will keep stealing electrons from other paired electrons until they are satisfied. This disrupts the normal chemistry of our cells and may lead to many health problems. Antioxidants (colorful fruits and vegetables, omega-3 fats, and green tea) give up or donate electrons to free radicals, thus quenching the free radicals' cravings. This is some of the science behind antioxidants and how they ward off cancer and heart disease and improve your health. Green tea is extremely high in antioxidants, helps boost the immune system, and aids digestion by improving the growth of beneficial bacteria in the intestines. Green tea has less caffeine than coffee and is more alkaline. Enjoy the wonderful health benefits tea may bring!

MILK

In the United States we drink over twenty-five gallons of milk per person per year. Of the milk we drink, over 90 percent is cow's milk. If you are currently drinking cow's milk, move to an organic source of cow's milk. As I mentioned earlier, the most consumed milk in the world is goat's milk! Okay, you may not be ready for goat's milk, but it is a healthy

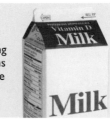

Many wonderful, great-tasting milk options are available to you.

option for those who may be allergic to lactose found in cow's milk. Goat's milk is easier to digest than cow's milk and contains caprylic acid, which is antifungal. Along with cow's and goat's milk, there are many wonderful, great-tasting milk options available to you. Oat milk, almond milk, hazelnut milk, rice milk, multi-grain milk, and soy milk are all plant-based milk options that taste great and are good for you. If you have problems with allergies, skin irritations, or respiratory issues, and like drinking milk, it may be time to look at the quantity and type of milk you are drinking. Almond milk is the most alkaline of your milk choices, followed by oat, rice, multi-grain, goat, soy, hazelnut, and cow's milk.

JUICE

As our lifestyles speed up, more and more people drink juice to get more fruits and vegetables into their diets. Drinking juice makes it easy to get a variety of valuable vitamins, minerals, and antioxidants. Juicing has become common practice for

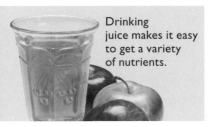

Drinking juice makes it easy to get a variety of nutrients.

many health-conscious consumers. Personally, I also find it challenging at times to get healthy nutrients into my body. I take wheat and barley grass juice daily in the form of a frozen ice cube. I just eat it like an ice cube or you can mix it with a cup of water. I take it first thing in the morning; it is easy, high in vitamins, minerals, and antioxidants, and is most al-

kaline. Believe it or not, it tastes good! Well, I like it. For many of my clients I also recommend diluting organic cranberry or pomegranate juice as a way to keep their bodies detoxified on a regular basis. Mix eight cups of water to one cup of organic cranberry or pomegranate juice, drinking one or two cups per day. I also add a shot of organic cherry juice to my mineral water; it is my evening cocktail. There is no substitute for eating whole fruits and vegetables, but drinking high-quality juice is the next best thing. When selecting juice choose only 100-percent, high-quality juice.

SPORTS DRINKS

Look for a sports drink that is high in electrolytes but does not contain high-fructose corn syrup.

One of the fastest-growing segments of the beverage industry is sports and energy drinks, especially with teenagers and young adults. It seems like everywhere you go, you see a sports or energy drink in the hand of these young people. In the gym, at a sporting event, or just hanging out, these drinks have exploded onto the beverage scene. Every major bev-

erage manufacturer now has its own line of sport and energy drinks. I think most people who use these products do not fully understand the impact these products have on the human body.

One ingredient that is highly prevalent in many beverages and processed foods is *high-fructose corn syrup.* Since the 1970s, when manufacturers began sweetening foods and beverages with high-fructose corn syrup instead of pricier sugar, Americans' consumption of the sweetener has skyrocketed, *a fact many researchers believe has been a major contributor to our dramatic rise in obesity, Type 2 diabetes, inflammation, heart disease, cancer, and mineral depletion.*

What makes high-fructose corn syrup so unhealthy? First, it is the amount of high-fructose corn syrup we consume. We are bombarded daily with high-fructose corn syrup. Manufacturers put this potent sweetener in everything from fast food to processed snacks and beverages. Second, in normal cell metabolism, insulin must be present to open up the cell to be fed. So, if you consumed a beverage that contained good old-fashioned sugar, your blood glucose would rise, insulin would be released, your cells would be fed, and your body would secrete the hormone leptin signaling satisfaction. Leptin is one of the hunger hormones that are released when the body is satisfied. High-fructose corn syrup can bypass normal cell metabolism, going directly into the cell so leptin is not released, and the body gets no indication that it is satisfied. This lack of satisfaction leads to greater consumption of the foods and beverages that contain high-fructose corn syrup.

I sometimes have to ask myself why a box of crackers, a bag of chips, or the hamburger bun at a fast-food restaurant contains high-fructose corn syrup in the first place. Does the product really need to be sweeter, or do manufacturers add high-fructose corn syrup to get you to eat more of their products? Take a look at your crackers, chips, peanut butter, soda pop, snack foods, and especially your beverages. *If high-fructose corn syrup is in the ingredient list, avoid that food or beverage!* You have an endless number of similar products to choose from that do not contain high-fructose corn syrup.

If you are engaging in endurance-type activities and are looking for a beverage that is high in electrolytes but does not contain high-fructose corn syrup, there are many drinks to choose from.

TAKE IT FROM ME...

Our personal training staff performs over 16,000 training sessions each year. We teach the principles talked about in *On Target Living Nutrition* on a daily basis and they have unquestionably changed the lives of thousands of our clients.

—Jason Block, Personal Training Director,
Michigan Athletic Club

ENERGY DRINKS

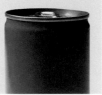

Most energy drinks are stimulants that can aggravate a number of health issues.

Another group of beverages that is growing extremely fast in popularity is energy drinks. What gives us the energy from the energy drink? That is a good question. Most of these high-octane drinks are loaded with caffeine and thermogenic compounds such as taurine, inositol, choline, and L-Carnitine. These thermogenic compounds are purported to produce heat and overstimulate the adrenal glands. Most of these drinks are stimulants that stress the adrenal glands, raise heart rate, elevate blood pressure, are extremely acidic, cause huge energy swings, deplete minerals, and may cause dehydration.

ALCOHOL

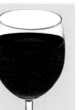

Red wine is the best choice if you wish to have an alcoholic beverage.

If you wish to drink an alcoholic beverage, is one better than another? Calories aside, red wine is your best choice. Red wine is not as acidic and has more antioxidants than other alcoholic beverages, followed by white wine, liquor, and beer. Beer is the most acidic alcoholic beverage. Drink alcohol in moderation.

WATER: YOUR BODY'S DRINK OF CHOICE

Water is essential for life and keeping the body healthy. The body is 70 to 75 percent water. Water is the body's cleansing and waste removal fluid. Water carries nutrients and oxygen, cushions joints, and protects organs. Water also aids in digestion and metabolism.

A common problem with many people is fatigue or lack of energy. Not having enough water contributes to fatigue. Water composes over 90 percent of your blood. As the body becomes dehydrated, blood is the first place your body looks for more water. When the body pulls water from the blood, blood volume decreases and your energy also decreases, due to a drop in cardiac output. From a health and performance standpoint, staying hydrated is critical!

Unintentional chronic dehydration may be the root of many serious diseases, including asthma, endocrine and kidney problems, high blood pressure, arthritis, ulcers, pancreatitis, digestive problems, low back pain, and obesity. A mere 2-percent drop in body water may lead to dizziness, fuzzy short-term memory loss, difficulty focusing, constipation, a drop in muscle contraction strength, and muscle cramping, as well as a drop in muscular endurance.

Keeping you body properly hydrated is not just about drinking the right amount of water. It is also important to understand water quality. The quality of the beverages we drink plays a huge role in balancing the body's pH level. Beverages such as alcohol, coffee, soda pop, energy drinks, and many sports drinks are acidic. As the acid levels in the body begin to rise, the body pulls out all of its defenses to bring pH back into balance. First, the body flushes the acid out of the body, causing greater dehydration. Second, valuable minerals such as calcium, magnesium, potassium, sodium, and iodine are slowly leached out of the body in an effort to buffer higher acid levels. Dehydration and many diseases, such as osteoporosis, high blood pressure, kidney stones, and Type 2 diabetes are linked to over-acidification of the body.

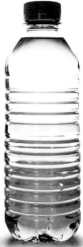

Is there a difference in types of water?

Okay, I understand the need to drink more water, but now you are telling me there are differences between the types of water we drink. I thought water was just water. Times have changed and so has the water we drink. Let's discuss the different types of water and determine the best type of water to drink.

Tap water

Many sources of tap water may contain chlorine and other toxic ingredients. Chlorinated tap water destroys beneficial bacteria in the body, which can weaken and damage the immune system. High levels of chlorine in drinking water have also been linked to heart disease and cancer. My first recommendation is to get your tap water checked for high levels of chlorine and other toxic ingredients. If you suspect your tap water to be unhealthy, you may want to look into buying an **ionized water filtration system.** Also, to improve the alkalinity of normal tap water, add a slice of lemon or lime.

Mineral water

One of the easiest ways to improve your health is to drink mineral water on a daily basis, twelve to twenty-four ounces a day. Mineral water is highly alkaline and helps to maintain essential minerals in the body. Choose only mineral water with naturally occurring carbonation. Mineral water can also be purchased without carbonation. In

Italy they say with or without the gas! So if you don't like mineral water due to the carbonation, you can purchase mineral water that has no carbonation. Add a slice of lemon or lime or a shot of juice for a refreshing taste.

Spring, artesian, or well water

Spring, artesian, and well water can all be excellent sources of drinking water. Spring water comes from an underground source that flows naturally to the earth's surface. Artesian water comes from a well that taps a confined aquifer, and well water comes from a manmade hole in the ground that taps an aquifer. All three sources are excellent for drinking. Store water in glass or inert plastic.

Purified or reverse-osmosis water

Creating "healthy water" means removing the harmful ingredients but keeping the beneficial minerals. Purified water sounds healthy, but is missing some important ingredients, namely minerals. Stripping the water of harmful toxins is good, but removing all the minerals from the water is not good. Drinking purified water over time can leach out valuable minerals from the body. Avoid drinking purified or reverse-osmosis water for any length of time.

Distilled water

More and more people are interested in the detoxification benefits of drinking distilled water. My recommendation is to increase the amount and quality of the water you drink and the body will naturally start to detoxify itself. *Do not drink distilled water on a regular basis because it draws minerals from the body and causes dehydration.*

Many bodybuilders drink distilled water two to three days prior to their contest in an attempt to rid the body of excess water and create the "ripped" look. Just last year one of the contestants I was competing against was so dehydrated he had to wait over five hours to come up with enough urine to be drug tested. I asked him later what he was doing to cause this excessive dehydration. He said he drank two gallons of distilled water two days in a row and then did not drink an ounce of water for the past two days. The only water he received was from the food he ingested. This may be an extreme case, but remember, distilled water is not to be ingested on a regular basis.

How much water do you need?

Ideally, you should drink half your body weight in ounces of water per day. If you weigh 150 pounds then you need approximately 75 ounces of water per day. *Your body's need for water increases with exercise.* Give your body the water it needs; let water be your drink of choice.

THE BOTTOM LINE

1. We are drinking more of our calories than ever before.
2. The number-one beverage consumed in the United States is soda pop, at seventy gallons per person per year.
3. Beverages such as soda pop, coffee, alcohol, distilled water, and energy drinks have high acidic levels and may lead to dehydration and mineral depletion.
4. Green tea is high in antioxidants, highly alkaline, and aids digestion.
5. Let water be your drink of choice, drinking approximately half your body weight in ounces of water per day. Store your drinking water in glass or inert plastic containers.

Recommended amounts of water per-day consumption

Weight	50% of weight or ounces of water	Approximate number of 16-oz. bottles or glasses of water
125 lbs.	63	4
150 lbs.	75	5
175 lbs.	88	5.5
200 lbs.	100	6
225 lbs.	113	7
250 lbs.	125	8
275 lbs.	138	8.5
300 lbs.	150	9

Chapter 14
THE KEY TO HEALTHY BONES

Americans have poor bone health when compared to people in other countries. The current recommendation for calcium intake in the United States is 1,000 milligrams per day for ages nineteen to fifty and 1,200 milligrams per day for ages fifty and over. The average American consumes 800 to 900 milligrams of

> The sun is always shining behind the clouds.

calcium per day, yet osteoporosis affects over 10 million American men and women. Approximately 50 percent of all women and 20 percent of all men over the age of sixty-five will experience bone fractures.

Countries such as Japan and Yugoslavia have a much lower intake of calcium—300 to 600 milligrams per day—and yet have a much lower incidence of osteoporosis. Countries with the highest intake of calcium—the United States, New Zealand, and Sweden—have higher, not lower, hip fracture rates.

People want healthy bones but don't always understand the impact their lifestyle plays on their bones. My daughter, Kristen, at age twenty-one, recently had her annual physical. The nurse asked Kristen how many glasses of milk she was drinking each day. Kristen said that she does not drink traditional cow's milk, she drinks soy milk. The nurse's response was, "Where are you getting your calcium from if you are not drinking cow's milk?" The nurse never asked Kristen if she was a soda pop or coffee drinker, was eating almonds, salmon, or green vegetables, and exercising regularly! I understand this way of thinking, but there is more to having healthy bones than just drinking cow's milk!

We have to understand two important factors that give us healthy bones. *First, buildup, what makes our bones strong? Second, breakdown, what makes our bones weak?* Much of our focus in the United States has been based on buildup, when in fact having healthy bones is a balance of buildup and breakdown.

WHAT WEAKENS BONES?

Lack of strength and balance exercises

As a society, we are just not getting enough exercise, especially strength and balance exercises. Many bone fractures are due to weak bones, but also due to poor balance leading to more falls. As we age, we need to stress the bones through exercise. This is one reason I recommend some form of strength training to almost everyone. We also lose our balance as we age; balance can easily be improved with a little practice. Many of my senior personal training clients tell me of situations in which they slipped and caught themselves. They truly believe if they had not been doing some strength and balance training they would have fallen and broken a bone. On pages 251–257 I have given you four to six exercises that will improve your balance, strength and flexibility, require no exercise equipment, and, best of all, take less than ten minutes to perform. Do you have ten minutes a day to improve your balance, strength, and flexibility? You don't have to spend hours in the gym to have healthy bones, but a little strength and balance training goes a long way to keeping your bones strong and your body healthy.

Acidosis and osteoporosis

Research links acidosis to osteoporosis. We now see low bone density (weak bones) in young women. There is a direct link between acid/alkaline balance and bone health. Bone is sensitive to small changes in blood pH. As the body becomes more acidic, pH levels change, with three bad results:

1. Mineral loss is increased.
2. Bone begins to break down.
3. Bone regeneration is inhibited.

Remember, you may be doing everything right to build your bones, but if you are leaching minerals out of the bones at a faster rate, you still may have weak bones.

What makes the body acidic?
Eating too much protein

If you weigh 150 pounds you only need 75 grams of protein. Getting more than 25 percent of your daily calories or more than a half a gram of protein per pound of body weight may cause the body to become overly acidic. This is one of the problems with many of the high-protein diets. Eating too much protein may lead to an unbalanced pH. When proteins break down, they must be neutralized by buffering minerals. If your protein intake is too high, buffering minerals from the bone may be depleted and a decrease of bone mass occurs.

High dietary intake of phosphate/phosphoric acid

Foods such as processed cheese, ice cream, artificial sweeteners, fried foods, beef, cocoa, sugar, table salt, pudding, lobster, cottage cheese, and any animal product that contains antibiotics create high acid levels in the blood. Beverages such as soda pop, coffee, beer, alcohol, and energy drinks also increase acid levels. The body must draw upon buffers to neutralize the excess acid. With the American teenager consuming three to six soda pops per day, it is easy to see why osteoporosis is now seen in young women and in some young men!

High levels of stress

Stress can eat up bones quickly. Stress triggers the hormones adrenaline and cortisol. Adrenaline and cortisol accelerate the acidity level of the blood, leading to mineral loss.

WHAT CAN YOU DO TO KEEP YOUR BONES HEALTHY?

Get adequate amounts of calcium and magnesium

Your recommended intake for calcium is 1,000 milligrams per day for adults up to age 50 and 1,200 milligrams per day for those over age 50. The recommended intake for magnesium is 420 milligrams per day for men and 320 milligrams per day for women. Magnesium is necessary for the secretion of the parathyroid hormone, which helps control the levels of calcium in the blood.

Food sources high in calcium and magnesium				
almonds	collard greens	oatmeal	soybeans	wheat and
amaranth	dairy products	parsley	spinach	barley grass
barley	figs	raisins	squash	
beans	kale	salmon	tofu	
broccoli	leafy greens	sardines		

Foods high in vitamin D	
cod liver oil	salmon
dairy products	sardines
free-range eggs	tuna
fortified whole-	
grain cereals	

Get enough Vitamin D

Vitamin D plays an important role in keeping your bones strong and healthy. Vitamin D helps your body utilize calcium. Recommended intake for Vitamin D is 600 to 800 units per day. Few foods naturally contain Vitamin D.

Getting fifteen to twenty minutes of natural sunlight increases Vitamin D production. Taking a multivitamin is also an easy way to get your daily requirement of Vitamin D.

Incorporate strength and balance exercises into your daily routine

Try to incorporate a five- to ten-minute strength and balance exercise program into your life. *See Chapter 26 to learn more about strength and balance.*

Eat and drink more alkaline-based foods and beverages

Fruits, vegetables, healthy fats, mineral water, green tea, sea salt, molasses, garlic, sweet potatoes, limes, lemons, watermelon, raspberries, cinnamon, sea vegetables, and pumpkin seeds all have high alkaline levels and help maintain alkaline/acid balance.

Avoid acid-based foods and beverages that are high in phosphates, phosphoric acid, and caffeine

Processed foods, soda pop, coffee, beer, table salt, cocoa, ice cream, fried foods, artificial sweeteners, and too much animal proteins are high in phosphates, phosphoric acid, caffeine, and arachidonic acid, which can lead to high acid levels in the body.

Control your stress

Some techniques to reduce your stress levels are deep-breathing exercises, positive self-talk, quiet time, meditation, yoga, exercise, soft music, a cup of herbal tea, a good night's sleep, or a brisk walk around the block.

TAKE IT FROM ME...

I think this is the greatest book I've read on nutrition and fitness. I've literally thrown out other books because they do not completely educate you on nutrition like this book does. I am eating nutritiously and well-balanced for the first time in my life. I've been trying to eat more nutritiously for many years, but I never realized what that fully meant, until I read this book.

Thanks for the section on "expect bumps in the road" because last week I fell off the wagon. The other night I sat down to reread some sections of your book and serendipitously I turned to the exact page with "Expect bumps in the road." I was feeling guilt and shame about some of my food choices over the past several days and needed the healthy encouragement. Now I feel re-energized!

—Holly Lehlbach

THE BOTTOM LINE

1. The United States has poor bone health when compared to other countries around the world.
2. Having healthy bones involves more than just consuming enough calcium.
3. Creating healthy bones is a balance between buildup and breakdown of our bones.
4. Many bone fractures are due to a lack of strength and balance in the body.
5. Consuming foods and beverages that are more alkaline and avoiding foods and beverages that are more acidic can directly improve the quality of bones and overall health.

TAKE IT FROM ME...

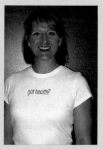

Rebecca Klinger

Through years of competitive figure skating, and a stressful, time-consuming career, I was an obsessive compulsive, people pleasing, perfectionist with a negative body image. I was continually searching for control through food restriction, purging, and obsessive daily rituals. Once diagnosed with clinical depression, I knew I needed a change. Unfortunately, my next career move would blindside me with a curve ball I never imagined. Within a year, I completely stopped exercising, began a love affair with Ben, Jerry, and Frito Lay, gained 43 pounds, and developed cancerous cells.

After treatment for the cancerous cells, I began a diet and exercise program. I lost some weight, but I continued to battle my depression, irritability, and fatigue for several more years, until I reconnected with Chris Johnson.

Progressing through On Target Living, Chris began showing me that true control was going to come from creating balance in my life. I began eating high-quality whole foods, and created a self-care environment by realistically decreasing work time, getting more sleep, and actually writing workout times into my schedule book. I am now three years into my On Target Living journey, and while I continue to be a people pleaser, the first person I try to please is myself. I physically and mentally feel the best I have ever felt. I have more energy, the tone of my self talk is more positive, and I feel much more comfortable in my own skin. I now spend my time living a well-balanced life. Oh! I almost forgot, there has been no return of the cancerous cells and I no longer have clinical depression.

An added bonus has been a dramatic improvement in the health of my parents and grandmother. While following the On Target Living plan, they have lost over 130 pounds and decreased the number of prescription medications used. Thank you, CJ, for inspiring three generations of our family.

Chapter 15
WHAT SHOULD YOU FEED YOUR KIDS?

A question regularly asked in my On Target Living seminars is, "What should I feed my kids?" I have twins, Kristen and Matt, who are in their twenties. Kristen and Matt are both healthy eaters and understand the benefits healthy eating brings. Living with "Mr. Granola" over the years, they probably didn't have much of a choice! From my own expe-

> In the middle of every difficulty lies opportunity.
>
> —Albert Einstein

rience, trying to get your kids to eat in a healthy way can be challenging and sometimes extremely frustrating. I would like to share with one of my earliest experiences in trying to shape my kids' nutritional patterns.

When Kristen and Matt were still in high chairs, I thought it would be a good idea for them to eat a healthier type of macaroni and cheese. Dinnertime can be a difficult time for parents and young children. Finding healthy foods that the kids like is hard. Kristen and Matt loved macaroni and cheese, so I decided to replace their usual macaroni and cheese with a healthier version (whole-grain macaroni and soy cheese). I figured if they didn't see me prepare the new version they wouldn't know the difference. Keep in mind that this was 1987 and at that time many of the so-called "health foods" didn't taste very good. When they first started to eat the macaroni and cheese, I was excited and smug, thinking my plan had worked. To my chagrin, both kids spit it out and started to cry after a few seconds of chewing. This was one of my first attempts to shape their nutritional patterns and I had failed miserably. But I learned a valuable lesson—nutritional changes need to be developed slowly for your kids, as well as for yourself.

With the explosion of refined foods and beverages, our kids are exposed to increasingly more unhealthy choices. Obesity, Type 2 diabetes, autoimmune diseases, poor bone health, allergies, fatigue, and attention deficit hyperactivity disorder (ADHD) have dramatically increased in our kids. If we think health care is out of control today, what do you think our health care is going to look like when our next generation of kids becomes adults?

Many schools are now getting on board offering healthier options in their cafeterias, but the greatest impact will come from home.

As parents, we want the best for our kids—we want them to develop into healthy, happy adults. When it comes to nutritional patterns, parents must set the tone. In my personal experience, *the best way to get your kids to eat healthy is for you to eat healthy!* Healthy nutritional patterns take time and energy to develop and require negotiation along the way.

TIPS TO GET STARTED

Tip #1: Improve food quality

Start by slowly cleaning out the refined foods in your house. What are some of the major food and drink items that your kids use on a daily basis? Soda pop, sports drinks, bread, chips, crackers, fast food, candy, peanut butter, hot dogs, macaroni and cheese, pizza, french fries, breakfast cereals, catsup. Start by improving the *quality* of these products. Down the road you may want to remove some of these products altogether, but start by improving the quality.

One thing I recommend to many parents is to improve the quality of peanut butter they are using from the refined, partially hydrogenated, unhealthy peanut butter to natural peanut butter. This is not a difficult change for most kids. Experiment with different brands of natural peanut butters. Not all taste the same. When you get the peanut butter home, stir it up, turn it upside down, and place it in the refrigerator. This keeps the peanut butter smooth and creamy. In most cases, within a week your kids will never miss the old, unhealthy version. Remember, partially hydrogenated or hydrogenated oils (trans-fats) make the cell membrane stiff and hard. Give your kids healthier options, especially for the foods they eat in larger quantities.

Current food item	Better choice
refined peanut butter	natural peanut butter
mayonnaise	canola mayonnaise
soda pop	water
french fries	make your own by baking with extra-virgin olive oil
sugared cereals	less refined cereals with added fruit
chips/crackers	snack foods with higher-quality fats
white bread	whole-grain bread
candy bars	energy bars
fruit juice	whole fruit

Tip #2: Be the leader

Practice healthy nutritional habits yourself. You set the tone and your kids will follow your lead. Give your kids a gift, the gift of good health. It's priceless!

Tip #3: Bring on the fat

Have your kids eat healthy fats every day. One of the healthiest things you can do for your kids is to give them a variety of healthy fats such as nuts, extra-virgin olive oil, natural peanut or almond butter, extra-virgin coconut oil, flax meal or flaxseed oil, and cod liver oil.

Tip #4: Place the food target on the refrigerator

Refer to the *Food Target* on a daily basis. Educate your kids about quality food choices from the *Food Target*.

Tip #5: Make small changes

Slowly replace unhealthy food and beverage choices. Don't try to change everything overnight. Be patient and build a strong foundation of healthy nutritional habits.

Tip #6: What's for dinner?

You don't have to be a short-order cook to keep everyone happy. Develop healthy mealtime habits and patterns and stick to your guns.

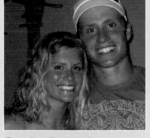

Our daughter and son, Kristen and Matt

Tip #7: Have healthy snacks available

Have easy, high-quality, accessible snacks around the house such as nuts, fresh fruit, organic chocolate milk, whole-grain cereals, whole-grain crackers, whole-grain bread, and natural peanut butter. Make your own smoothie drinks for after-school snacks and for before and after sporting activities.

Tip #8: Develop a team approach

Work with your kids. Educate them. Discuss with them what they like. Give them options that you both can agree on. Take them to the grocery store. Create a team approach to healthier nutrition.

One book I highly recommend for getting your kids to eat healthy is *Baby Bites* by Joann Bruso (www.babybites.info).

These are just a few ideas to get you started. Educate your children, be patient, and lead by example. Help them recognize the benefits of eating healthy. And don't worry when they say, "There's nothing to eat in the house!" They won't starve.

THE BOTTOM LINE

1. To get your kids to eat healthier, you must eat healthier. Be the leader!
2. Start slowly and make small changes.
3. Help to educate your kids on making better nutritional choices.
4. Bring on the fat! Get healthy fats into your kids' nutritional program.
5. Make healthy snacks readily available to your kids.

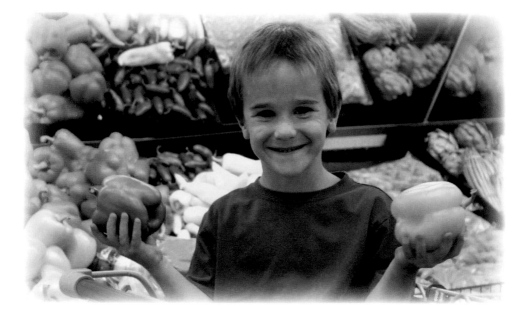

steps to success

Chapter 16
PUTTING IT ALL TOGETHER

Now that you have come this far, you have the nutritional knowledge to succeed, but as we all know in life it takes more than just knowledge to be successful. Successful change also requires that you think about whether you are *ready* to make changes, *what* changes you want to make, *why* you want to make those changes, and *how* you will make the changes happen so you get what you want.

> ## Change starts when someone sees the next step.
> —William Drayton

This section is about *taking action*. Begin your action plan at your own pace. Research shows that small changes are more successful than multiple behavior changes all at once. Baby steps are the key; otherwise, it can be overwhelming.

Recently a man approached me after one of my seminars and asked if it would be possible to get off his addiction to the soft drink Mountain Dew™. I asked him "How many Mountain Dews™ are you drinking per day?"

He replied, "Nine." I thought to myself, "Now that is a lot of Mountain Dew™."

What do you think would have happened if I had suggested drinking green tea or a shot of wheat grass juice to replace his Mountain Dew™? I think he would have run for the hills! I suggested he cut back to five or six Mountain Dews™ per day for the first month and start drinking mineral water with lemon or a shot of juice to add a little flavor. Six months later, I received an email beaming that he is completely off his Mountain Dew™. Sometimes people are ready to change and he obviously was.

If you want to start with one small step like eating one fruit a day or drinking more water, great. If you are ready to make multiple changes, it's up to you; you are the driver of this bus! One small step leads to the next step, which leads to more. Take the first step and don't look back. Now let's get busy and take some action.

MAKING THE DECISION TO CHANGE

The first step is to decide! Are you ready to make some changes in how you think, feel, and act about lifestyle choices you are currently making? You might read this book and find a few small things you want to change or, perhaps, you have already made some changes and are ready to take it to the next level. Making the decision to change is your first step to a healthier way of life. Just do it! Make a change!

WHAT DO YOU WANT TO CHANGE?

Take some time now to sit down, think, and decide *what you want to change* about your current lifestyle. Is your goal to become healthier, leaner, stronger, and to have more energy? Your answer becomes your destination, the focus of your action plan.

WHY DO YOU WANT TO CHANGE?

Next, decide *why you want to change.* The "why" question is everything! After one of my seminars, a woman introduced herself to me and told me that she had weighed over 300 pounds three years ago and today she weighs 140 pounds. Wow! She was beaming from ear to ear and full of energy. Many people in the crowd overheard her story and, of course, wanted to know how she did it.

> Nothing is impossible to a willing heart.
>
> —John Heywood

After congratulating her on wonderful success and sharing some of the strategies she had used, I had to ask the question, "Why did you want to change?"

She said, "I knew you would ask me that question. One day while staying with my granddaughter, I found her crying in her bedroom, so I asked her, 'Honey, why the big tears?' My granddaughter responded, 'Grandma, I am afraid you won't live long enough to attend my high school graduation.' It was like someone had stuck a knife in my heart! Right then and there, I had my why."

The "why" behind the change is extremely powerful. The why is your source of motivation to do the hard work of replacing old habits with new habits. What do you want for your life? What roses do you want to smell in your future? Why do you want to change? **Put your back-burner dreams on the front burner!**

PLAN TO SUCCEED AND SUCCEED WITH A PLAN

Planning plays a critical role in successfully developing healthy lifestyle habits. This is the "how" question. In our fast-paced lives, it can be difficult to eat as healthy as you would like, especially when you get busy or while traveling. It is easy to get out of your normal routines, and this is when you may get into trouble.

What should you do if you feel yourself sliding backwards or having trouble just getting started in your quest for better balance, energy, and vitality? I believe one of the real keys to success is developing action plans so your behaviors become daily rituals. Rituals become a part of you, like taking a shower or brushing your teeth, lifestyle habits that you don't really have to think about. When I asked this question of you, it made me think, "What rituals do I have? How dialed-in is my hierarchy of human needs? Is my dog, Dolly, better at this than I am?" There are a few rituals I do on a daily basis, whether I am at home, working, or traveling.

First is rest and recovery! I focus on two areas of rest and recovery—sleep and deep breathing. I focus on getting a minimum of six hours of sleep per night. Ideally, seven to eight hours is my plan, but at times, six hours is all that I get. Taking short, one-minute deep breathing breaks is another way to help rejuvenate myself throughout the day.

Second is exercise! I do a combination of yoga poses that takes only five to seven minutes, and walk or climb stairs. Both can be done almost anywhere. My target exercise program is more involved, but on some days, it just doesn't work. Move your body daily!

Third is nutrition! Staying properly hydrated each day is a major focus. I drink a minimum of eighty ounces of water plus twelve to sixteen ounces of mineral water per day. My goal is 100 ounces, but 80 ounces of water is something I do every day. I also consume wheat grass, flaxseed oil, cod liver oil, organic extra-virgin coconut oil, and extra-virgin olive oil each day. I also eat at least one big salad full of greens and vegetables. Oh, I almost forgot! A day rarely goes by without some form of oatmeal and fruit for breakfast. I like the taste and the steady energy it gives to the start of my day.

To help you on your way to healthier nutritional rituals, here are some suggestions for actions you may want to include in your nutrition action plan.

Food preparation

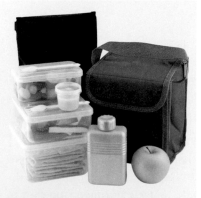

Plan ahead, pack your favorites

One of the keys to consistently eating healthy is food preparation. I rarely leave the house without packing a few meals or snacks, especially if I am going to be gone for the entire day. On a typical day I pack water, oatmeal, fruit, and a big salad with leftovers from the night before (chicken, baked yams, and broccoli, for example). I usually pack all my food and beverages the night before. This takes me less than ten minutes and allows me to eat and drink frequent, high-quality meals and snacks throughout the day, keeping me satisfied and feeling great!

The excuse I commonly hear from personal training clients or seminar attendees is, "I don't have time to make breakfast or prepare foods and beverages for the day." If mornings are too busy for food preparation, take ten minutes the night before and pack healthy foods for the next day. It doesn't take long to get your food and beverages ready, but it does take a commitment to change some of your daily habits. With a little planning you can have healthy, energy-sustaining foods and beverages at your fingertips.

Developing daily rituals or habits is the essence of *On Target Living Nutrition*. If planning your entire day nutritionally seems too overwhelming in the beginning, then start with breakfast. For those of you who think you don't have time for breakfast, mix up a smoothie or "oatmeal on the run" the night before. They taste great and get your day off to a great start.

One key for quick food preparation is to have the right equipment on hand. Here are a few equipment suggestions that will help in your success in eating healthier:

- **Small cooler and plastic containers:** A small cooler is great for taking food or beverages to work or travel. I use a soft cooler with plastic containers to carry my breakfast, snacks, lunch, and beverages every day. I never leave home without it!
- **Blender:** A blender is great for mixing up smoothie drinks and other recipes like oatmeal pancakes.
- **Toaster oven:** Excellent for heating up leftovers and browning vegetables or anything that needs to be heated up in a hurry.
- **Food steamer:** It's great for steaming vegetables, potatoes, eggs, rice, and oatmeal.
- **Juicer:** A juicer can be an excellent way to get more fruits and vegetables into your diet. I juice wheat grass in my juicer every few weeks. I buy the wheat grass from the health food store, cut the grass, place it in the juicer, pour the juice into ice cube trays, and freeze the juice. It is a convenient way for me to get fresh wheat grass juice into my diet on a daily basis.

Decide what you want to eat for breakfast, snacks, lunch, and dinner for the next few days or week

Scan your house and work environment. Then go shopping. Experiment with foods you like and make them easy to eat. I enjoy a big salad for lunch, so I buy bags of prewashed organic spinach or romaine lettuce, broccoli, slaw, and sprouts and throw them into a large resealable plastic bowl. I add Alaskan salmon, tuna, or a chicken breast, walnuts, dried cherries, and a dressing of extra-virgin olive oil and balsamic vinegar. This takes me less than five minutes to prepare. I take this to work or toss it together at home for a fast, easy, healthy meal.

Keep quick and easy food sources in the house or at work

Good staples include mineral water, spring water, fresh fruit, celery, carrot sticks, nuts, eggs, whole-grain cereals, whole-grain or sprouted bread, whole-grain crackers, energy bars, natural peanut or almond butter, and organic yogurt, to name a few.

Plan for eating on the run

When you travel, you don't have to cave in to unhealthy eating practices. Organic whole food bars, bottled water, dried fruit with nuts, and a balanced smoothie drink are all fast and convenient ways to maintain your energy and vitality. When you travel, plan ahead. See Chapter 24, "Healthy Eating on the Run," for more information.

Develop new daily rituals

Where can you make improvements? Take some time to prepare food for the next day or your entire week. Her are a few easy options to choose from:

- extra chicken breasts
- sweet potatoes
- oatmeal on the run
- smoothies
- hard-boiled eggs
- salad bar in the fridge
- baked vegetables
- homemade soup
- your favorite leftovers

Spend ten minutes the night before and get ready for your day

Your action plan is your road map for change. Be sure that your action plan includes how to get support from family and friends, how you will record your progress, how you will overcome roadblocks to success, and the behaviors that are specific and realistic for *you* to do. Your action plan depends on you. Where are you starting from and where do you want to go? How much change are you ready to make? Remember, many of my rituals are fairly new to me. Forty years ago I was eating Captain Crunch™ cereal for breakfast and a bologna sandwich on white bread with mayo served with Beefaroni™ for lunch! Your goal is to develop a few lifestyle rituals of your own. Focus on one or two specific areas you want to improve upon—no different than brushing your teeth or taking a shower.

Changing your old rituals takes extra time and effort in the beginning. Chapters 17 to 26 will give you even more ideas to help you develop your action plan. Remember, the rewards for better health, energy, and vitality are priceless!

TAKE IT FROM ME...

On Target Living has played an integral part in my personal and professional life. I have used the various knowledge and principles from Chris Johnson to increase the quality of my clients' health and fitness goals. I feel that Chris has done his homework and has brought such a powerful and life-changing book to the top of the industry. I have helped people of all ages, from young to old, to top athletes using Chris's On Target Living information. This book has brought my training and nutrition principles to the next level.

—Justin Grinnell, Personal Trainer, East Lansing, Michigan

THE BOTTOM LINE

1. Make the decision to change.
2. Decide what you want to change and why you want to change.
3. Develop your realistic and specific action plan— your road map:
    • Get support from family and friends.
    • Record your progress.
    • Overcome roadblocks.
    • Outline behaviors you will start and behaviors you will stop doing.
4. Do your action plan.
5. Continue to tweak your action plan until healthier choices become rituals.

Chapter 17
WRITE IT DOWN

When people consult with me about personal training or have questions concerning weight loss or health issues, I usually ask them to fill out a food log for two or three days. I think many people are apprehensive at first because they don't understand the importance of fueling their bodies. By monitoring your daily eating, drinking, activity, and sleeping habits and recording them in a daily food log, you can usually find areas in which you can make improvements. The food log is an awareness tool to help you determine where you are and the changes you may want to make.

> The shell must break before the bird can fly.
> —Alfred, Lord Tennyson

Not long ago I received a food log from a woman who wanted to lose weight. She had been fighting this battle for many years. She was eating approximately 1,200 calories per day and exercising six days a week for sixty to seventy-five minutes, and was extremely frustrated by her inability to lose weight. From looking at her food log, I could see she needed more balance in her plan. She was sleeping less than five hours per night, drinking too much coffee and diet pop, eating low-quality foods, and consuming few healthy fats. She spent most of her days thinking about food and weight loss.

So we sat down and started from the beginning. We discussed getting healthy at the cellular level first. *Our entire discussion focused on food quality, not calories or quantity.* I wanted her to quit counting calories. I wanted her to focus on improving her food quality. She learned how to use the *Food Target* to help her guide her choices. Along with improving her food quality she added a little healthy fat to each meal, increased her frequency of eating, added four one-minute deep-breathing breaks during the day, and improved the efficiency of her exercise program in the morning, which allowed her to get more sleep. At first, she thought she was not exercising enough to lose weight. I encouraged her to focus on the quality of her exercise program, not on quantity. She improved her posture during her exercise program and throughout her day. She slowly began to shift her attention to getting healthy, not to losing weight. She was getting excited about the thought of getting fit. Within six weeks she was beginning to see changes in her energy, hair, skin, and mood, and her pants were feeling loose. She was feeling good. She started to truly believe her body was working with her, not against her. The momentum of developing healthy lifestyle habits was taking shape, and she was ecstatic.

In her case the daily food log was an extremely valuable tool in helping her understand where she was and the changes she needed to make. Losing weight is not just about eating less and exercising more. A daily food log is one tool that can help you look at the big picture of health.

HOW TO USE THE DAILY FOOD LOG

Write down the time of each meal. Under description, write what you ate and the approximate serving size. Place a check inside the *Food Target* to represent a carbohydrate, protein, or fat. Many foods you choose will be a combination of all three macronutrients. Remember that the most nutritious, nutrient-dense foods are closer to the center of the target, the green area of the *Food Target*. At the bottom of the daily food log, indicate the amount of water you drank, hours of sleep, and kinds of physical activities you performed, and then write a brief description of your thoughts, feelings, and energy level during the day. The daily food log is a learning tool that you can use over and over.

THE BOTTOM LINE

1. Use the daily food log as a learning tool.
2. Use the daily food log to monitor your food and beverage consumption, sleep, physical activity, thoughts, feelings, and physical well-being.
3. Use the daily food log to determine what areas need improvement and focus on making the necessary changes.
4. Use the daily food log as a tool to get back on track if you find yourself starting to drift from your plan.
5. Focus on quality first!

Sample Food Log		
Day: Thursday	Date: June 7, 2007	
MEAL	DESCRIPTION	TARGET
Breakfast Time: 6:30	oatmeal (2/3 cup) soy milk dried organic cherries slivered almonds lemon-flavored cod liver oil	
Snack 1 Time: 10:00	CJ's smoothie (water, flaxseed oil, banana, frozen berries, hemp protein powder)	
Lunch Time: 12:00	big salad (spinach and Romaine lettuce, broccoli slaw, walnuts, sliced strawberries, tuna in water, balsamic vinegar and extra-virgin olive oil)	
Snack 2 Time: 2:45	organic low-fat cottage cheese frozen blueberries lemon-flavored cod liver oil	
Dinner Time: 6:00	salmon fillet baked yams kale, onion, garlic, extra-virgin olive oil	
Snack 3 Time: 9:30	toasted slice of sprouted bread organic extra-virgin coconut oil mineral water	

Water (8 oz.)	☑ ☑ ☑ ☑ ☑ ☑ ☑ ☑ ☐ ☐ ☐
Sleep (hours)	4 ☐ 5 ☐ 6 ☐ 7 ☐ 8 ☑ 9 ☐ 10 ☐
Activity/exercise	☑ Cardio ☑ Strength ☑ Flexibility ☐ Other
Breathing breaks	☑ ☑ ☑ ☐ ☐ ☐ ☐ ☐ ☐ ☐
Meditation/napping	☐ ☐ ☐ ☐ ☐ ☐ ☐ ☐ ☐ ☐
Comments	Great day! Energy was high, sleep was restful.

Chapter 18
HOW TO READ A LABEL

For many people, reading food and beverage labels can be confusing—fat-free, low carbs, cholesterol-free, high-protein, organic, zero trans-fats, 100-percent natural. Food and beverage manufacturers can make it extremely difficult to determine the quality of what you are consuming. When you look at a food or beverage label, what you see is not always what you get. How do you know if a food or beverage is healthy?

> All of the significant battles are waged within the self.
>
> —Sheldon Kopp

Reading a food label does not have to be confusing any more. Here are seven questions to ask yourself that will help you have a better understanding of food labels.

HOW LONG IS THE INGREDIENT LIST?

If you learn one thing about understanding food labels this is it—*less is best!* Generally, the shorter the ingredient list the healthier the food or beverage. If you pick up two different loaves of bread, bags of chips, bottles of salad dressing, boxes of breakfast cereal, or frozen pizzas and place them side by side, you can quickly determine which of the two products is healthier solely by the number of ingredients listed on the label. For example, a typical loaf of refined white bread may have over forty-five ingredients, whereas a loaf of sprouted whole-grain bread may have fewer than eight ingredients. You won't see an ingredient list on fresh fruits or vegetables. These products are in their natural state. Remember when looking at a food label, less is best!

Let's compare two breakfast cereals, 100-percent rolled oats (oatmeal) and Blueberry Crisp™. The oatmeal has only one ingredient, 100-percent rolled oats. Oatmeal is nutrient-dense, high in fiber, has a better balance of

Oatmeal

INGREDIENTS: 100% ROLLED OATS

Blueberry Crisp Cereal

INGREDIENTS: CORN, SUGAR, BLUEBERRIES (BLUEBERRIES, HIGH FRUCTOSE CORN SYRUP, GLYCEROL, SAFFLOWER OIL, CITRIC ACID, CALCIUM LACTATE, POTASSIUM SORBATE [PRESERVATIVE], NATURAL BLUEBERRY FLAVORING), ROLLED OATS, SLICED ALMONDS, PARTIALLY HYDROGENATED SOYBEAN AND/OR COTTONSEED OIL, SALT, HONEY, MALT EXTRACT, RICE, PARTIALLY HYDROGENATED SUNFLOWER OIL, HIGH FRUCTOSE CORN SYRUP, NATURAL AND ARTIFICIAL FLAVOR, NONFAT MILK, MOLASSES, CORN SYRUP
VITAMINS AND MINERALS: SODIUM ASCORBATE AND ASCORBIC ACID, NIACINAMIDE, FERRIC ORTHOPHOSPHATE, PYRIDOXINE HYDROCHLORIDE, VITAMIN A PALMITATE, RIBOFLAVIN, THIAMIN HYDROCHLORIDE, FOLIC ACID, VITAMIN D.

carbohydrates, proteins, and fats, has no unhealthy fats, no added sugar or artificial ingredients, will maintain a steady blood glucose level, and is extremely inexpensive. Contrast this with the Blueberry Crisp™ cereal, which has a long ingredient list, contains high-fructose corn syrup, artificial ingredients, and trans-fatty acids, and is more expensive.

Natural Dressing

INGREDIENTS: EXPELLER PRESSED CANOLA OIL, WATER, CIDER VINEGAR, BUTTERMILK POWDER, ORGANIC SUGAR, SEA SALT, EGG POWDER, ONION POWDER, GARLIC POWDER, XANTHAM GUM.

Refined Dressing

INGREDIENTS: SOYBEAN OIL, WATER, VINEGAR, SUGAR, EGG YOLKS, SALT, CONTAINS LESS THAN 2% OF WHEY, ONIONS*, BUTTERMILK, MONOSODIUM GLUTAMATE, XANTHAM GUM, PHOSPHORIC ACID, WITH SORBIC ACID AND CALCIUM DISODIUM EDTA AS PRESERVATIVES, GARLIC*, POLYSORBATE 60, PARSLEY*, SPICE, NATURAL FLAVOR *DRIED

DO YOU RECOGNIZE ALL THE WORDS IN THE INGREDIENT LIST?

The ingredient list starts with the most predominant ingredient by weight, and continues in descending order. In the next example, we compare two types of ranch salad dressing. Ranch dressing A has a much shorter ingredient list, higher-quality ingredients, and contains no added preservatives. Ranch dressing B has a longer ingredient list, poor-quality ingredients, and contains an unhealthy food additive, monosodium glutamate (MSG). Once you understand the labels, choosing dressing A is easy.

WHAT IS THE SERVING SIZE?

When looking at any label, always check the serving size or number of servings in the product. How many times have you reached into a bag of chips and thought nothing of it? After a closer look at the serving size (one ounce or approximately seven chips equals 140 calories) you may have exceeded the serving size and then some. I know I have! Three or four handfuls of chips, and the next thing I know I have consumed over 400 calories of chips! Be aware that calories can add up quickly if your serving size exceeds the label recommendation.

Also be aware that manufacturers can label products low-fat, light, fat-free, or trans-fat free based on a serving size. If a product has less than 0.5 grams of fat per serving, the Food and Drug Administration (FDA) will allow that product to be labeled fat-free or trans-fat free, even if the product is 100-percent fat! For example, extra-virgin olive oil (C) is 100 percent fat, with fourteen grams of fat per tablespoon. Compare that to the same brand of extra-virgin olive oil no-stick cooking spray (D), which claims to be free of fat, calories, and cholesterol. This labeling is based on less than 0.5 grams of fat per serving. In this example, a serving size of the no-stick spray is one-third of a second or less. I have tried this many times and have found it impossible to spray the pan for only one-third of a second! So if you use the spray for one-third of a second or less, It is labeled fat-free, but what if you use it for a full three seconds? Read the label and note the serving size.

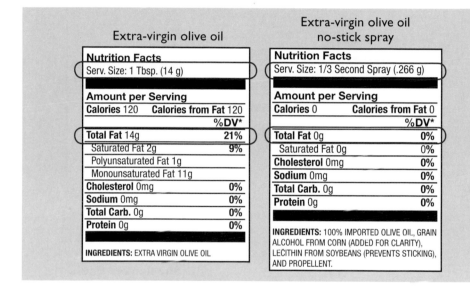

WHAT KIND OF FAT?

It is important to learn how to distinguish healthy fats from unhealthy fats with the goal of eliminating trans-fats from your diet. Trans-fats are in any product that lists hydrogenated or partially hydrogenated oils. Be aware that "no trans-fats" on a label does not always indicate that the product is free of trans-fats! According to FDA labeling regulations, a product can claim to be trans-fats free if it contains less than 0.5 gram per serving. *If you see hydrogenated or partially hydrogenated in the ingredient list, the product contains trans-fats!*

To become your healthiest, eliminate refined saturated fats and fractionated oils as well. Fractionization is a process that removes some of the more saturated fats. This keeps a product from thickening or freezing when stored in a cool place. *Search for healthy fats such as unrefined saturated, monounsaturated, and polyunsaturated (omega-3 and omega-6) fats.*

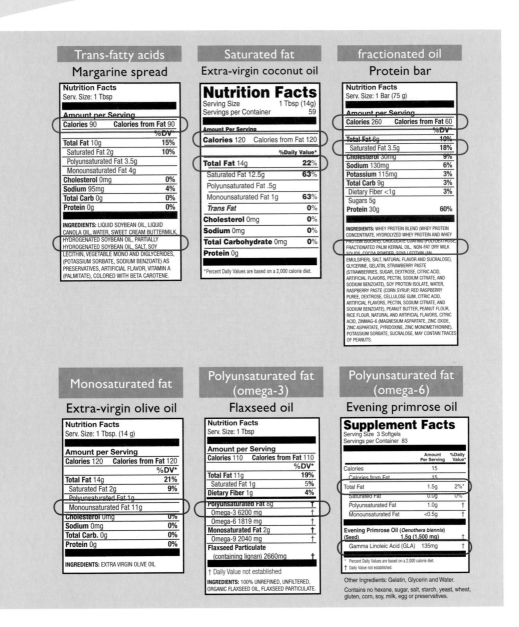

WHAT TYPE OF SWEETENER?

There are many different sweeteners that manufacturers are now using and many of these sweeteners are camouflaged as something other than sugar. Avoid foods or beverages with high-fructose corn syrup, corn syrup, sucrolose, dextrose, or any artificial ingredients, such as aspartame. In most cases added sweeteners are refined.

You are better off buying foods and beverages that are not sweetened. Add your own sweeteners such as organic sugar, honey, or molasses, and if you don't want the spike in your blood glucose, your best choices are stevia and agave nectar.

WHAT IS THE BALANCE OF CARBOHYDRATE, PROTEIN, AND FAT?

First, determine the number of grams of the nutrient you are calculating.

Second, multiply the number of grams by the number of calories per gram. This will equal the calorie content of that nutrient in the product.

Third, divide the calories of that nutrient by the total calories in the product per serving, which will equal the percent of that nutrient in the product.

Calories per gram	
I gram of fat = 9 calories	I gram of protein = 4 calories
I gram of carbohydrates = 4 calories	I gram of alcohol = 7 calories

EXAMPLE: Raisin Bagel

Use the final calculation to determine the proportion of each of the macronutrients within the total calories:

Step 1

Total calories = 230
Total FAT = 2.5 grams
Total CHO = 44 grams
Total PRO = 8 grams

Step 2

2.5 grams × 9 calories = 22.5 calories from FAT
44 grams × 4 calories = 176 calories from CHO
8 grams × 4 calories = 32 calories from PRO

Step 3

22.5 FAT calories ÷ 230 total calories = 10% FAT
176 CHO calories ÷ 230 total calories = 77% CHO
32 PRO calories ÷ 230 total calories = 14% PRO

HOW WAS THE FOOD OR BEVERAGE GROWN OR PROCESSED?

You may want to buy foods that are free of antibiotics, pesticides, and chemicals. Look for products labeled 100-percent organic. For more information on buying organic, go to Chapter 6, "Going Organic."

THE BOTTOM LINE

1. Less is best when looking at the number of ingredients in a food label.
2. If you don't recognize words in the ingredient list, beware!
3. Pay attention to serving sizes.
4. Avoid foods and beverages that contain partially hydrogenated or hydrogenated oils, artificial sweeteners, and high-fructose corn syrup.
5. Focus on improving the quality of your foods and beverages.

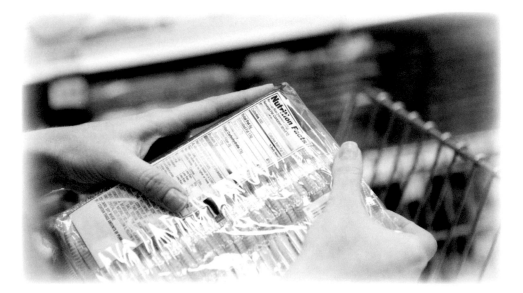

Chapter 19

SHOPPING 101

When you fill your shopping cart wisely, you are well on your way to a healthier you. If you have unhealthy food in your house, clean out your pantry and refrigerator and start fresh. Almost all of your healthier food and beverage items can be purchased in most conventional grocery stores. Many have a natural or organic food section. I would also recommend that you find a natural food store in your area. Most have a large selection of natural food and beverage items and a knowledge-able staff.

> There is never a traffic jam on the extra mile.

Below is a suggested shopping list. I have listed many items, but this is by no means exhaustive. Experiment and ask questions. Remember that shopping is a learning process and can be enjoyable. Go with a plan of action—make a list.

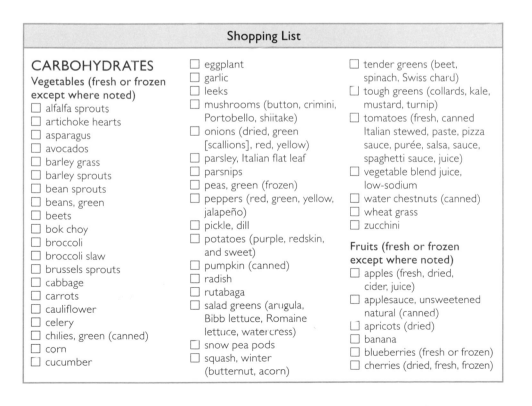

Shopping List

CARBOHYDRATES
Vegetables (fresh or frozen except where noted)
- ☐ alfalfa sprouts
- ☐ artichoke hearts
- ☐ asparagus
- ☐ avocados
- ☐ barley grass
- ☐ barley sprouts
- ☐ bean sprouts
- ☐ beans, green
- ☐ beets
- ☐ bok choy
- ☐ broccoli
- ☐ broccoli slaw
- ☐ brussels sprouts
- ☐ cabbage
- ☐ carrots
- ☐ cauliflower
- ☐ celery
- ☐ chilies, green (canned)
- ☐ corn
- ☐ cucumber

- ☐ eggplant
- ☐ garlic
- ☐ leeks
- ☐ mushrooms (button, crimini, Portobello, shiitake)
- ☐ onions (dried, green [scallions], red, yellow)
- ☐ parsley, Italian flat leaf
- ☐ parsnips
- ☐ peas, green (frozen)
- ☐ peppers (red, green, yellow, jalapeño)
- ☐ pickle, dill
- ☐ potatoes (purple, redskin, and sweet)
- ☐ pumpkin (canned)
- ☐ radish
- ☐ rutabaga
- ☐ salad greens (arugula, Bibb lettuce, Romaine lettuce, watercress)
- ☐ snow pea pods
- ☐ squash, winter (butternut, acorn)

- ☐ tender greens (beet, spinach, Swiss chard)
- ☐ tough greens (collards, kale, mustard, turnip)
- ☐ tomatoes (fresh, canned Italian stewed, paste, pizza sauce, purée, salsa, sauce, spaghetti sauce, juice)
- ☐ vegetable blend juice, low-sodium
- ☐ water chestnuts (canned)
- ☐ wheat grass
- ☐ zucchini

Fruits (fresh or frozen except where noted)
- ☐ apples (fresh, dried, cider, juice)
- ☐ applesauce, unsweetened natural (canned)
- ☐ apricots (dried)
- ☐ banana
- ☐ blueberries (fresh or frozen)
- ☐ cherries (dried, fresh, frozen)

Shopping List *continued*

☐ cherry juice
☐ cranberries (dried)
☐ cranberry juice
☐ dates (dried)
☐ grapes (red and green)
☐ kiwi
☐ lemons (for zest and juice)
☐ lime (for zest and juice)
☐ mandarin oranges (canned)
☐ mango
☐ oranges
☐ orange juice
☐ peaches
☐ pears
☐ pineapple (fresh, canned)
☐ pomegranate juice
☐ prunes (dried)
☐ raisins (dried)
☐ red raspberries
☐ strawberries (fresh, frozen)

Cereals/Breads/Grains
☐ barley, pearled
☐ breads (buns/rolls, lavash, pita, pizza crust, whole wheat, sprouted grain)
☐ bulgur
☐ cereal, Ezekiel 4:0 Original™
☐ cereal, Uncle Sam™
☐ cookies, chocolate wafer, natural
☐ cornmeal
☐ flour, whole grain unbleached, unbromated (wheat, rice, oat…)*
☐ noodles, whole grain
☐ oat bran
☐ oats, rolled
☐ pasta, whole grain (capellini, couscous, lasagna, macaroni, noodles, penne, spaghetti, vermicelli…)
☐ quinoa
☐ rice, brown, long-grain
☐ rice, mixed wild
☐ rice cakes, whole grain
☐ rice protein powder
☐ tortilla chips (high-oleic safflower oil or expeller-pressed canola oil)

☐ Wasa™ crackers
☐ wheat gluten

Beans/Legumes
☐ beans (black, cannellini, garbanzo, great northern, kidney, navy, pinto, red, refried [fat-free, canned], white)
☐ hummus (prepared)
☐ lentils

PROTEINS
Meat/Poultry/Fish
☐ beef (sirloin, tenderloin, flank steak)
☐ buffalo (ground, medallions, roast, steak)
☐ chicken breast, boneless/ skinless
☐ chicken thighs (bone-in, boneless)
☐ clams (canned)
☐ cod, wild-caught
☐ crab
☐ ostrich, ground
☐ pork (loin chops, tenderloin)
☐ red snapper
☐ salmon, wild-caught
☐ scallops
☐ shrimp
☐ tuna fish, wild-caught (canned in water)
☐ turkey (ground breast, whole, ham [uncured, nitrate and nitrite-free], deli slices)
☐ venison, ground, steaks

Eggs/Dairy
☐ butter, organic
☐ cheese, organic, low-fat (cheddar, cottage, feta, pepper, Monterey jack, mozzarella, ricotta, swiss, Parmesan)
☐ cream, sour (organic, low-fat)
☐ eggs, organic, free-range
☐ goatein powder

☐ milk, organic (canned fat-free evaporated, non-fat dry powder, skim [almond, goat, oat or rice milk can be substituted in recipes for cow's milk])
☐ protein powder (hemp, rice, soy, whey)
☐ yogurt, organic, low-fat (plain and flavored)

Soy
☐ milk, soy
☐ milk, soy (carob)
☐ Soy Delicious Frozen Dessert® (chocolate velvet)
☐ tofu, firm

FATS (UNREFINED)
Nuts and Seeds
☐ almond butter*
☐ almonds, raw (sliced or slivered)
☐ Brazil nuts
☐ flax meal*
☐ flaxseeds, whole
☐ hazelnuts
☐ peanut butter, natural (smooth or crunchy)*
☐ peanuts
☐ pine nuts
☐ pumpkin seeds
☐ sunflower seeds
☐ walnuts*

Oils
☐ almond oil
☐ canola oil, expeller-pressed
☐ canola oil mayonnaise
☐ coconut oil, extra-virgin, unrefined
☐ cod liver oil, lemon-flavored
☐ Earth Balance® spread*
☐ flaxseed oil*
☐ macadamia nut oil
☐ olive oil, extra-virgin, unrefined
☐ sesame oil, toasted*

Shopping List *continued*

Other
- [ ] avocado
- [ ] olives, green and ripe

HERBS/SPICES/ CONDIMENTS
- [ ] allspice
- [ ] anchovy paste
- [ ] barbecue sauce
- [ ] basil, sweet (dried or fresh)
- [ ] bay leaves (dried)
- [ ] Bragg Liquid Aminos™
- [ ] capers
- [ ] chili powder
- [ ] chives, fresh
- [ ] cilantro
- [ ] cinnamon (ground, stick)
- [ ] cloves
- [ ] coriander
- [ ] cumin, ground
- [ ] dill (dried or fresh)
- [ ] garlic powder
- [ ] ginger
- [ ] gingerroot (fresh)
- [ ] hoisin sauce
- [ ] horseradish
- [ ] hot pepper sauce
- [ ] Italian herb mix
- [ ] lemon pepper

- [ ] marjoram (dried or fresh)
- [ ] mint, fresh
- [ ] mustard (regular, Dijon and dry)
- [ ] nutmeg, ground
- [ ] onion powder
- [ ] oregano (dried or fresh)
- [ ] oyster sauce
- [ ] paprika
- [ ] parsley, Italian flat leaf
- [ ] peach chutney
- [ ] pepper, cayenne
- [ ] pepper, red (flakes)
- [ ] pepper, black (peppercorns)
- [ ] poultry seasoning
- [ ] rosemary
- [ ] rum extract
- [ ] sage
- [ ] savory (dried)
- [ ] sea salt
- [ ] sea salt based seasoning salt
- [ ] shoyu sauce
- [ ] soy sauce, reduced-sodium
- [ ] steak sauce, organic
- [ ] stir-fry sauce
- [ ] tamari sauce
- [ ] tarragon
- [ ] teriyaki sauce
- [ ] thyme (dried or fresh)

- [ ] vanilla extract, pure
- [ ] wine (dry white, rice)
- [ ] Worcestershire sauce

MISCELLANEOUS
- [ ] agar powder
- [ ] arrowroot
- [ ] baking powder, aluminum-free
- [ ] baking soda
- [ ] bouillon, chicken, low-sodium
- [ ] broth, low-sodium (beef, chicken, fish, vegetable)
- [ ] chocolate, bittersweet baking
- [ ] chocolate chips, organic
- [ ] cocoa powder, unsweetened
- [ ] maple syrup
- [ ] sweeteners (honey, Stevia Plus™ blend, brown and granulated sugar)
- [ ] vinegars (balsamic, apple cider, red wine, rice, tarragon)
- [ ] water (spring, artesian, mineral)

*Store whole-grain flours, unrefined oils, ground flaxseeds, and raw nuts in refrigerator to protect against rancidity and nutrient loss. Whole-grain flours can also be frozen to protect freshness.

THE BOTTOM LINE

1. Get a fresh start by cleaning out your refrigerator and cupboards.
2. Find a grocery store that fits your needs. If they don't have what you are looking for, ask.
3. Go with a plan. Sit down and make a list. Don't go shopping when you are hungry.
4. Spend most of your time shopping on the outer perimeter of the store. This is where your healthiest food choices are displayed.
5. Find a natural, organic foods store in your area.

Chapter 20

THE THREE-HOUR RULE

The first thing most people do when they want to lose weight is cut calories. Most people believe the easiest way to decrease calories is to skip meals. Unfortunately, this is just the opposite of what you need to do. Skipping meals slows down your metabolism. This is just one reason why eating breakfast is so critical to your success. It is important to break the overnight fast and fuel the body properly. Along with a slow metabolism,

> The only time you can't afford to fail is the last time you try.
>
> —Charles Kettering

skipping meals alerts the body to release more of the fat-storing enzyme, lipoprotein lipase. Lipoprotein lipase becomes more sensitive when meals are skipped. It's one of the body's safety mechanisms to protect against starvation. Remember, skipping meals is a strategy used by sumo wrestlers to gain weight!

If one of your goals is to rev up your metabolism, then increase the frequency of your meals and spread your calories throughout the day, I call this **"The Three-Hour Rule."** Ideally, try to eat every three hours. By eating more frequently, you will:

- Increase your metabolic rate, allowing you to burn more calories.
- Improve energy by maintaining a steadier blood glucose level.
- Make better food choices because you won't be as hungry.
- Control portion sizes more easily

During the first few weeks, make small changes. Eat the same foods and quantities, but eat more frequently. If you find yourself eating one large meal per day, move to two meals per day. Try not to eat more than 600 to 800 calories at any one meal. If you are eating three good-sized meals per day, move to four meals per day. If you want a higher metabolism, increased energy, and better health follow **The Three-Hour Rule.**

The chart on the next page shows a comparison of how meals can be spaced throughout the day, with a progression from poor to best.

There will always be days when you will find it difficult to eat every three hours. Plan ahead and remember that enjoying fresh fruit and a few nuts, or a smoothie drink is an easy way to improve your frequency of eating.

POOR 2,000 calories	GOOD 2,000 calories	BETTER 2,000 calories	BEST 2,000 calories
6:30 a.m. skip	6:30 a.m. 400 calories	6:30 a.m. 350 calories	6:30 a.m. 350 calories
noon skip	noon 700 calories	9:30 a.m. 250 calories	9:30 a.m. 250 calories
7:00 p.m. 2,000 calories	7:00 p.m. 900 calories	noon 500 calories	noon 450 calories
		3:30 p.m. 250 calories	3:00 p.m. 200 calories
		7:00 p.m. 650 calories	6:00 p.m. 600 calories
			8:00 p.m. 150 calories
I meal	3 meals	3 meals, 2 snacks	3 meals, 3 snacks

THE BOTTOM LINE

1. Most people skip meals to cut calories.
2. Lipoprotein lipase is a fat-storing enzyme that becomes more sensitive when meals are skipped.
3. One of the sumo wrestlers' strategies to gain weight is to skip meals.
4. Always eat breakfast!
5. By eating frequent, small meals, you improve your metabolism, energy, portion control, and health. Use The Three-Hour Rule.

Chapter 21

IT'S QUALITY, QUALITY, QUALITY

We all know the old adage when buying real estate, it's "location, location, location." Throughout this entire book you have heard me stress quality, quality, quality.

> We cannot direct the wind...
> but we can adjust the sails.

Quantity is important and I will get to that, but I want to begin with quality. Personally, when I look back over the years, the thing that has changed the most in my own nutritional plan is the quality of foods and beverages I use. I am always trying to improve the quality of nutrients that I am consuming. Nutrients such as wheat grass, barley grass, mineral water, parsley, purple potatoes, organic game meats, organic extra-virgin coconut oil, and sea vegetables are relatively new to my nutritional plan. You may be thinking, "Who eats wheat grass, sea vegetables, and organic game meats?"

As I mentioned earlier, most diet programs focus on quantity or calories first. Cutting calories and exercising more is the strategy most people take to lose weight. Yes, you may lose weight in the beginning, but can you sustain this type of plan, and second, are you healthy at the cellular level? My primary goal is to get you to think about making small changes and improving the quality of the food and beverages you are consuming. For example, if you enjoy peanut butter on a piece of toast for breakfast, then focus on improving the quality of the peanut butter and the quality of the bread. You may add or delete foods or beverages down the road, but first focus on improving quality. Remember, one of your first goals is to get healthier at the cellular level, not deprive the body of calories.

INCREMENTAL CHANGES

Take small steps when improving your nutritional plan. Over time, these small steps become a permanent part of your routine. Do you remember Mikey in that old Life Cereal™ commercial: "Give it to Mikey, he won't eat anything." Mikey was a finicky eater, and then Mikey takes a bite and likes it. People seldom like a new taste or texture the first time they try it, especially if they think it is good for them. When switching from two-percent milk to skim or soy milk, many people do not like the initial change, but within a week or so they get used to it and then they start to like it.

A question I hear in many of my seminars is, "How does it taste?" Whenever I talk about cod liver oil and its wonderful health benefits, most people get this disgusted look on their faces! For years, I have been trying to get some of my family members to start taking cod liver oil. The cod liver oil is lemon-flavored and tastes like a lemon drop, honestly. I knew how the cod liver oil could improve their health, so at Christmas a few years ago I poured everyone a shot of cod liver oil. (Don't you wish you could spend Christmas at my house?) Most thought it tasted okay, not as bad as they anticipated, and many decided this was something they could do. My mom now preaches the benefits of cod liver oil and its refreshing taste to anyone who will listen.

Do you choose foods that taste good or foods that are good for you? Can you have foods that are good for you and taste good

Many people have a difficult time understanding how wheat grass or lemon-flavored cod liver oil is part of my daily routine. Maybe my taste buds were out to lunch the first time I tried them. My intention was not that these products were going to taste good; my intention was that I wanted the wonderful health benefits that they bring.

too? Absolutely! But you need to be willing to try new tastes and textures and be patient. Many people have a difficult time understanding how wheat grass or lemon-flavored cod liver oil is part of my daily routine. Maybe my taste buds were out to lunch the first time I tried them. *My intention was not that these products were going to taste good; my intention was that I wanted the wonderful health benefits that they bring.* I remember the first time I tried wheat grass. It was not something I was extremely fond of, but over time I actually grew to like the unique grassy taste. I think I lost some credibility with that statement. Honestly, I look forward to taking my wheat grass every morning. It has a clean taste and I truly believe my energy has improved by taking it. Improving the quality of the foods and beverages you eat and drink makes a tremendous difference in how you look and feel and in your overall health.

To improve the quality of your food or beverages, be conscious of what you buy at the grocery store. Read labels and buy foods in their most natural state. Let's see how you can improve the quality of your food over time. I'll use myself as an example. When I was in college, my typical breakfast was:

CJ's breakfast thirty years ago
- Sugared cereal
- Two-percent milk
- Refined white bread toast with butter
- Orange juice

Compare that breakfast—full of refined carbohydrates, with minimal protein and no healthy fats—with today's breakfast.

CJ's breakfast today
- Frozen wheat grass and water
- Organic rolled oats
- Organic soy milk
- Flaxseed oil
- Cod liver oil
- Slivered almonds
- Organic dried cherries

This transition happened slowly. I experimented with foods and gradually improved the quality of the carbohydrates, proteins, and fats in my diet. With each change, I enjoyed more satisfaction, greater energy, and a better mood throughout the day. I also enjoy this breakfast. I can't imagine reverting to my old college breakfast. If you told me thirty years ago that I would be eating wheat grass, uncooked oatmeal, soy milk, flaxseed oil, cod liver oil, slivered almonds, and organic cherries I would have said, "No way. Are you nuts?"

Steps to improve breakfast		
Week 1	Week 2	Week 3
2 cups of coffee	1 cup of coffee	1 cup of green tea
cream (for coffee)	skim milk (for coffee)	½ whole-grain bagel
bagel	½ bagel	natural peanut butter
cream cheese	natural peanut butter	½ orange or ½ cup berries
	½ orange	2 free-range organic eggs
	water	water

Let's look at some incremental steps you can take to improve the quality of your food.

Now look at some similar progressions for lunch, whether you are eating out or packing your lunch. We'll incorporate small, steady changes and show the progress from week one through weeks six and twelve.

In any of these examples, the timing may be faster or slower depending on your goals and your choices.

Improving the quality of your food can be challenging. With the prevalence of convenience and fast foods, it is easy to eat calorie-dense foods that are low in quality and low in nutritional value. The more refined the food, the lower the quality. Be prepared to shop smarter and look for quality in the foods you choose. Make special requests when you are dining out to get exactly what you want.

Steps to improve lunch—eating out		
Week 1	Week 6	Week 12
hamburger	broiled chicken sandwich	chicken breast
french fries	side salad	vegetables
	fat-free vinaigrette	2 small redskin potatoes
		extra-virgin olive oil on potatoes
diet soda pop	water	water

Steps to improve lunch—brown bag		
Week 1	Week 6	Week 12
white bread	enriched white bread	whole-grain bread
packaged lunch meat	deli turkey	organic turkey breast
mayonnaise	fat-free mayonnaise	canola mayonnaise
candy bar	iceberg lettuce	romaine lettuce, slice of tomato
	applesauce	apple
soda pop	juice drink	water

The chart below shows how to progress from low-quality to higher-quality foods.

Poor	Better	Best
margarine	butter	organic butter
olive oil	virgin olive oil	extra-virgin olive oil
refined peanut butter		natural peanut butter
iceberg lettuce		romaine lettuce, spinach
whole milk	skim milk	organic skim milk, soy, rice, oat
fried chicken	baked chicken thighs	organic baked chicken breast
juice drink	fruit juice	whole fruit

QUANTITY—CALORIES DO COUNT!

Now that you have a better understanding of food and beverage quality, it is time to turn our attention to quantity. You can consume the right kinds of foods and beverages, but if you consume too much at any one time (gorging), or over the course of the day, week, month, or year, one or more of these problems may arise:

- overproduction of insulin
- drop in energy
- imbalance of hormones
- increased body fat
- poor health

How many calories should you consume each day?

The number of calories you need to eat and drink each day depends on many factors, such as your activity level, lean muscle mass, stress, frequency of meals, and food and beverage quality.

Activity level: How much exercise do you get each day? How sedentary is your lifestyle? Is your job physical? How active is your day? Do you routinely walk, bike, hike, climb stairs, strength train, dance, or do yoga?

Lean muscle mass: The more lean muscle mass you have, the more calories your body burns at rest and throughout the day. There are over ten times more mitochondria in a muscle cell than a fat cell. So to keep your body burning calories, keep your mitochondria healthy and active. This is one reason strength training is so important in maintaining your metabolism.

Stress: Don't underestimate the role of stress and its effect on how many calories you need. Stress is vital for keeping us at the top of our game, but too much stress can lead to overeating—and the release of the stress hormone cortisol. Too much cortisol can break the body down and may lead to an increase in body fat.

Frequency of meals: When you eat more frequently (three-hour rule), your body uses the food more efficiently, making it more difficult to overeat or drink.

Food and beverage quality: High-quality carbohydrates, proteins, and fats along with quality hydration keep the body running at its peak.

Your daily calorie needs may vary, depending how you day unfolds. Try to listen to your body and its nutritional needs. If you are truly hungry, eat. But challenge yourself first—are you truly hungry, or just bored or stressed and looking for some relief? It will take time to develop new nutritional patterns. Below is a range of calories to work with. Remember, this is just a range. Your goal is not to count calories, but you must be conscious of the quantity of food and beverages you consume and this gives you a starting point.

Your body needs quality food and water in adequate amounts in order to stay healthy and to feel your best. You may exceed the high-end calorie range based on your activity level, lean muscle, stress level, and frequency and quality of meals. Lumberjacks have been known to consume over 11,000 calories per day in an attempt to maintain their body weight. Because there are many variables when it comes to how many calories you need per day, these ranges are just guidelines. Listen to your body and its nutritional needs.

> Calorie ranges per day
> Adult female: 1,200–2,100
> Adult male: 1,500–2,500

How many calories should you consume at each meal?

This may vary depending on the time of day, the last time you ate, or when you will eat next. Eating more than 600 to 800 calories per meal, depending on your nutritional needs, may be too many calories. I have done this a few times, especially at Thanksgiving. The average amount of calories consumed on Thanksgiving Day is over 5,000 calories! I can't throw stones at this number. I know I have been part of this crowd on more than a few occasions and, boy, do I feel lousy afterwards!

Eating high-calorie meals may lead to high insulin levels, poor energy, increased fat storage, and unbalanced hormone levels. Your goal is to spread your calories over the course of the day, with breakfast, lunch, and dinner comprising your larger meals, and inserting small snacks in between.

Calories per meal over the course of a day			
	1,200 calories	1,800 calories	2,500 calories
breakfast	250 calories	325 calories	450 calories
snack	100 calories	150 calories	250 calories
lunch	350 calories	500 calories	650 calories
snack	100 calories	150 calories	250 calories
dinner	400 calories	550 calories	700 calories
snack		125 calories	200 calories
Total	1,200 calories	1,800 calories	2,500 calories

Understanding serving sizes

The best laid plan for healthy eating can be negated if you are unaware of how much you are eating. A few years ago, while monitoring my own nutritional program, I was surprised at how many calories I was consuming per day! I was eating fairly high-quality foods spread over the course of the day, but was not as lean as I wanted or expected to be. So, for three days, I filled out a food log, analyzed my meal plans, and converted each meal and snack into specific calorie counts. I was shocked at my overall calorie intake, especially at breakfast. My breakfast consisted of oatmeal, soy milk, raisins, and walnuts. I have been eating oatmeal for breakfast since my grandmother turned me on to it when I was just a small child. (My grandmother lived to the ripe old age of ninety-eight, and she grew up eating oatmeal.) My food quality was healthy; I was just eating too much, 875 calories of oatmeal, nuts, raisins, and soy milk is too much for breakfast! I just cut my portions in half and substituted slivered almonds for the walnuts. My calorie count for breakfast went from 875 to 360 calories.

By the way, this oatmeal recipe is not cooked and is served cold. I place all the ingredients in a small bowl in the refrigerator overnight. The milk soaks in, the flavors mix, and in the morning I have a great-tasting, healthy breakfast.

	Old breakfast		Improved breakfast	
oatmeal	1½ cups	450 calories	⅔ cup	200 calories
almonds	2 tbs.	240 calories	sprinkle	60 calories
raisins	⅛ cup	65 calories	handful	40 calories
soy milk	10 oz.	120 calories	5 oz.	60 calories
Total		875 calories		360 calories

TAKE IT FROM ME...

It was after I had my second son that I received Chris Johnson's first book, *Meal Patterning*, in a completely random way. I was on the Body For Life forum on the website, and I had posted something about working on my terrible addiction to sugar. Someone replied asking for my address to send me a copy of a book that had helped them. I gave him my address, and he sent me the book. I still wasn't really ready to make the major changes necessary to get me on track, so it sat on my shelf for some months until my mom was visiting. She picked it up to flip through it and told me it was pretty good. So I started reading it and changed my eating habits pretty much immediately. I feel like I just didn't know how to make better choices than I was making at the time, which is what I encounter now in my students as a yoga and pilates instructor.

People really want to do better, but it is really hard to sort the good information from the bad. I recommend this book every chance I get. I tell people there are four moments in my adult life that have left the most profound imprints. They are meeting my husband, the birth of my first son, receiving this book, and meeting my yoga teacher. *Meal Patterning* had an immeasurable deep effect on my life. I basically took my bodyfat from a post-pregnancy high of 30 percent down to 15 percent with the knowledge gained from the book and regular exercise. I am truly grateful to have found this book when I did and to have the opportunity to instill healthy eating habits in my two children.

—Leanna Williams, Yoga and Pilates Instructor, Houston, Texas

The Carpenter and the Contractor

An elderly carpenter was ready to retire. He told his employer-contractor of his plans to leave the house-building business and to live a more leisurely life with his family. He would miss the paycheck, but he needed to retire. The contractor was sorry to see his good worker go and asked if the carpenter could build just one more house for him as a personal favor. The carpenter said yes, but in time it was easy to see that his heart was not in his work. He resorted to shoddy workmanship and used inferior materials. It was an unfortunate way to end his career. When the carpenter finished his work and the contractor came to inspect the house, the contractor handed the front-door key to the carpenter. "This is your house," he said, "my gift to you." What a shock! What a shame! If he had only known he was building his own house, he would have done it all so differently. Now he had to live in the home he had built none too well.

So it is with us. We build our lives in a distracted way, reacting rather than acting, willing to put up with less than the best. At important points we do not give the job our best effort. Then with a shock we look at the situation we have created and find that we are now living in the house we have built. If we realized that, we would have done it differently.

Think of yourself as the carpenter. Think about your house. Each day you hammer a nail, place a board, or erect a wall, build wisely. It is the only life you will ever build. Even if you live it only for one day more, that day says, "Life is a do-it-yourself project." Your life today is the result of your attitudes and choices in the past. Your life tomorrow will be the result of your attitude and the choices you make today.

—Author Unknown

QUICK-PICK FOOD LIST

To speed up the process of understanding serving sizes, the quick-pick food list will help you create a serving size image. This will allow you the to look at a food item and estimate the serving size and its approximate calories.

CHO (Carbohydrates)

VEGETABLES
1 cup = 8–15 grams = 32–60 calories
asparagus
mushrooms
zucchini
cucumbers
green, red, yellow bell peppers
brussels sprouts
green beans
broccoli
spinach
kale
cabbage
onions
romaine lettuce
peas (½ cup)
carrots (½ cup)
corn (½ cup)
potato (1 medium = 20 grams of CHO =
   80 calories)
yam (1 medium = 20 grams of
   CHO = 80 calories)

FRUITS
20 grams = 80 calories
apple (1 medium)
grapefruit (1 medium)
nectarine (1 large)
peach (1 large)
apricot (4 fresh)
dates (4 pitted)
green grapes (¾ cup)
sweet cherries (¾ cup fresh)
blackberries (1 cup)
cantaloupe (1½ cups)
red raspberries (1½ cups)
strawberries (1½ cups)
watermelon (1¾ cups)
banana (1 small= 25 grams of CHO = 100 calories)
kiwi (2 = 25 grams of CHO = 100 calories)
raisins (2 tbs.)
dried cherries (2 tbs.)

CEREALS, GRAINS, LEGUMES
30 grams = 120 calories
black beans (½ cup)
garbanzo beans (½ cup)
lentils (½ cup cooked)
bagel (½)
cooked cereal (½ cup)
cold cereal (½ to 1 cup)
flour tortilla (1)
pita bread (1½ slices)
whole-grain bread (1½ slices)
rye bread (2 slices)
brown rice (1 cup cooked)
pasta (1 cup cooked)
puffed wheat (2 cups)

Note: Many of these carbohydrates also contain protein.

QUICK CONVERSIONS
⅛ teaspoon	a pinch
1 tablespoon	3 teaspoons
⅛ cup	2 tablespoons
¼ cup	4 tablespoons
⅓ cup	5½ tablespoons
½ cup........8 tablespoons	4 ounces
1 pint	2 cups
1 quart	4 cups
1 gallon	4 quarts
1 ounce	2 tablespoon
28.3 grams	1 ounce

More Conversions
1 gram of carbohydrate	4 calories
1 gram of protein	4 calories
1 gram of alcohol	7 calories
1 gram of fat	9 calories

Stevia Plus™ to Sugar
Stevia Plus	Sugar
1 packet	2 tsp.
¼ tsp.	1 tsp.
2 tbs.	½ cup

QUICK-PICK FOOD LIST CONTINUED

Note: Meat, fish, and eggs also contain fat, but do not contain carbohydrates. Dairy, soy, and grains contain carbohydrates and some fat. Most protein powders contain little if any carbohydrate unless they have been sweetened.

PROTEINS

MEAT
30 grams = 120 calories
skinless chicken breast (4 oz.)
skinless turkey breast (4 oz.)
venison (4 oz.)
buffalo (4 oz.)
ostrich (4 oz.)
lean pork (4 oz.)
lamb (4 oz.)
flank steak (3 oz.)

FISH
30 grams = 120 calories
salmon (4 oz.)
tuna (4 oz.)
cod (4 oz.)
shrimp (6 oz.)

EGGS, DAIRY
free-range eggs (1 egg white = 6 grams of protein)
feta cheese (¼ cup = 6 grams of protein)
part-skim mozzarella cheese (¼ cup = 6 grams
    of protein)
low-fat cottage cheese
    (½ cup = 13 grams of protein)
nonfat yogurt (1 cup = 12 grams of protein)
skim milk (1 cup = 8 grams of protein)

PROTEIN POWDERS
1 tablespoon = approximately 15–17 grams
of protein
whey
soy
goat
rice
hemp

SOY
soy nuts (1 oz. = 12 grams of protein)
tofu (3 oz. = 6 grams of protein)
tempeh (½ cup = 15 grams of protein)
soybeans (½ cup = 14 grams of protein)
soy milk (1 cup = 7 grams of protein)

FATS

1 tbs. = 13 grams = 120 calories

TRANS-FATTY ACIDS*
hydrogenated or partially hydrogenated oils
margarine
shortening

SATURATED
organic butter
organic extra-virgin coconut oil

MONOUNSATURATED
canola mayonnaise
extra-virgin olive oil
almond oil
olives
avocados
natural peanut butter
slivered almonds
almond butter

OMEGA-3
flax meal
flaxseed oil
fish oils
cod liver oil
walnuts
most nuts

OMEGA-6
evening primrose oil
sunflower oil
pumpkin seed oil
sesame oil

*eliminate or minimize these fats in your diet

THE BOTTOM LINE

1. Focus on food and beverage quality first.
2. Use the *Food Target* to help guide your selections
3. The amount of calories you need depends on your activity level, lean muscle mass, stress, frequency of meals, and food quality.
4. It is important to understand serving sizes so you don't overeat.
5. To speed up the process of understanding serving sizes, use the quick-pick food list in helping you create a serving size image.

TAKE IT FROM ME...

As a previous Crimfit participant, I was fortunate to participate in one of Chris Johnson's On Target Living seminars and had the opportunity at that time to purchase Chris's book. I am another "success story." Due to Chris Johnson and his book, I was able to reduce my cholesterol by sixty points in less than six months without medications.

—Marjorie Figg

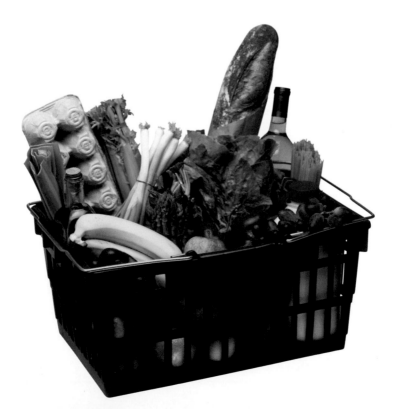

Chapter 22

BALANCING THE "BIG THREE"

Is it really necessary to get a balance of carbohydrates, proteins, and fats at every meal? How specific or accurate does this balance need to be? What will happen if I eat just carbohydrates or just proteins or just fats? These are some of the questions I receive in regards to getting the ideal balance of the three macronutrients in your nutritional program.

> What wisdom can you find that is greater than kindness?
>
> —Jean-Jacques Rousseau

First, is it necessary to get a balance of carbohydrates, proteins and fats at each meal? Ideally, yes! This may not always happen, but having balance is the target you are aiming for. The body needs a balance of the three macronutrients to perform at its best. If for breakfast you start your day with only carbohydrates but little or no protein and fat, it makes it difficult to get all the proper nutrients to keep your body healthy. It's the combination that makes the body function at its best.

Second, do you have to be specific or accurate in balancing the three macronutrients? No, just try to get in the ballpark. I have given you some guidelines to follow in balancing your carbohydrates, proteins, and fats. Get a little of each macronutrient at most of your meals and snacks. It may be as simple as changing from your fat-free salad dressing at lunch to adding extra-virgin olive oil for more balance.

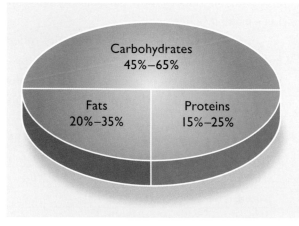

Adding a few nuts to your breakfast cereal or adding a small piece of fish or chicken to your favorite salad are just a few examples of ways you can create more balance to your meals. I want you to be aware of your balance, but I also want you to make it simple!

Third, there will be situations where you won't have an opportunity to balance your meals or snacks. Is it okay to eat just an apple, a salad, a few nuts, or a piece of chicken? Absolutely, but eating a piece of chicken with sliced apple in a salad and a few nuts will give your body a greater variety of the nutrients it needs for greater health and performance. Do the best you can with what's available.

Sample breakfast—poor balance, poor quality			
	Carbohydrate	Protein	Fat
coffee	0 g	0 g	0 g
sugared cereal	45 g	2 g	1.5 g
whole milk	12 g	8 g	8 g
2 slices toast w/margarine	40 g	2 g	12 g
Totals 630 calories	97 g 388 calories	12 g 48 calories	21.5 g 193.5 calories
Balance	61% CHO	8% PRO	31% FAT

BREAKFAST

In the example above, there are too many calories, refined carbohydrates (sugared cereal, white bread), poor-quality fats (whole milk, butter), and little protein. Let's make it better.

Start by replacing sugared cereal with rolled oats. Switch from whole milk to soy milk (you'll be surprised how good soy milk tastes). Eliminate the white bread. Add raisins for increased potassium and fiber. Finally, add high-quality fat (walnuts). There are fewer calories, more vitamins, fiber, and high-quality foods.

Sample breakfast—improved balance, good quality			
	Carbohydrate	Protein	Fat
water	0 g	0 g	0 g
rolled oats	27 g	4 g	3 g
soy milk	6 g	6 g	3 g
raisins	15 g	0 g	0 g
walnuts	2 g	2 g	7 g
Totals 365 calories	50 g 200 calories	12 g 48 calories	13 g 117 calories
Balance	55% CHO	13% PRO	32% FAT

LUNCH

Sample lunch—good balance, poor quality			
	Carbohydrate	Protein	Fat
tuna	0 g	22 g	I g
white bread	20 g	2 g	I g
light mayonnaise	0 g	0 g	10 g
salad	22 g	2 g	I g
fat-free dressing	18 g	0 g	0 g
diet pop	0 g	0 g	0 g
Totals 461 calories	60 g 240 calories	26 g 104 calories	13 g 117 calories
Balance	52% CHO	23% PRO	25% FAT

In the example above, we have poor-quality carbohydrates and fats and very low nutritional value. Let's make a few changes.

Sample lunch—good balance, good quality			
	Carbohydrate	Protein	Fat
tuna	0 g	22 g	I g
salad	22 g	2 g	I g
sliced strawberries	20 g	0 g	0 g
balsamic vinegar and extra-virgin olive oil	2 g	0 g	10 g
slivered almonds	4 g	4 g	5 g
water with lemon	0 g	0 g	0 g
Totals 457 calories	48 g 192 calories	28 g 112 calories	17 g 153 calories
Balance	42% CHO	25% PRO	33% FAT

We have improved all areas of this lunch; first, by eliminating the white bread and mayonnaise, and second, by replacing the fat-free dressing with balsamic vinegar and extra-virgin olive oil (good fats). We added sliced strawberries and slivered almonds for more fiber, vitamins, and minerals. We replaced the diet soda pop with water and a slice of lemon. This lunch has higher-quality foods, and is healthier, more satisfying, and more energy-sustaining.

DINNER

We can show the same improvements in a dinner meal.

Sample dinner—poor balance, poor quality			
	Carbohydrate	Protein	Fat
beef tips/gravy	0 g	46 g	30 g
noodles	30 g	4 g	2 g
two rolls with butter	35 g	4 g	20 g
corn	35 g	4 g	2 g
fat-free frozen yogurt	25 g	2 g	0 g
diet soda pop	0 g	0 g	0 g
Totals 1,226 calories	125 g 500 calories	60 g 240 calories	54 g 486 calories
Balance	40% CHO	20% PRO	40% FAT

Any time you eat this many calories (1,226) and an overabundance of refined carbohydrates (noodles, rolls, and frozen yogurt) at one meal, your insulin levels will skyrocket and fat storage is inevitable. This meal has too many refined carbohydrates, too much protein, and its fat content is primarily from saturated fats. There's just too much food. Let's see how we can clean this meal up.

Sample dinner—improved balance, good quality			
	Carbohydrate	Protein	Fat
flank steak	0 g	30 g	6 g
two redskin potatoes	30 g	1 g	0 g
1½ cups asparagus	20 g	1 g	0 g
1 tbs. extra-virgin olive oil	0 g	0 g	10 g
water	0 g	0 g	0 g
Totals 472 calories	50 g 200 calories	32 g 128 calories	16 g 144 calories
Balance	42% CHO	27% PRO	31% FAT

Start off by replacing the beef tips with flank steak, which is very lean and tastes great. Then substitute redskin potatoes and asparagus for the refined carbohydrates (noodles and rolls) and replace the butter with extra-virgin olive oil. Once again, notice the substitution of water for soda pop. The result: a healthy, balanced, great-tasting meal with 754 fewer calories.

SNACKS

The same balance should apply to your daily snacks.

Sample snack—poor balance, poor quality			
	Carbohydrate	Protein	Fat
pretzels	25 g	1 g	1 g
diet soda pop	0 g	0 g	0 g
Totals 113 calories	25 g 100 calories	1 g 4 calories	1 g 9 calories
Balance	88% CHO	4% PRO	8% FAT

With this snack, we once again see a high percentage of carbohydrates, low protein, and low fat. It's poorly balanced and consists of poor-quality foods. This snack will do little to support your energy or your health. Let's make it better.

Sample snack—improved balance, good quality			
	Carbohydrate	Protein	Fat
smoothie drink	24 g	11 g	6 g
Totals 194 calories	24 g 96 calories	11 g 44 calories	6 g 54 calories
Balance	49% CHO	23% PRO	28% FAT

This is a great snack for breakfast, at work, while traveling, or after your workout. With this balanced drink, you get quality carbohydrates, protein, and fat for only 194 calories in a twelve-ounce drink. See the recipe section for other smoothie recipes.

Consider substituting higher-quality foods in any meal or snack. Even dessert presents an opportunity to improve the balance and quality of your foods.

CJ's special smoothie

Makes three 12-oz. servings

3 cups water
1 banana
2 scoops hemp or rice protein
   powder
1½ tbs. flaxseed oil
1 bag frozen unsweetened berries
   (16 oz.)

Put all ingredients in blender and mix about one minute. Keep refrigerated.

THE BOTTOM LINE

1. **Get balanced:** Ideally, try to get a balance of carbohydrates, proteins, and fats throughout your day.

2. **Macronutrient ranges:** Carbohydrates: 45–65 percent, proteins: 15–25 percent, fats: 20–35 percent. Use these ranges as guidelines.

3. **You don't have to be exact:** Don't make yourself crazy trying to get the correct balance. Try to get a little of each of the three macronutrients at most meals and snacks.

4. **Be aware of your nutritional balance each day.** Be aware of your nutritional balance when eating. Do you have high-quality carbohydrates, proteins, and fats?

5. **Stand-alone meals:** There will be situations in which you won't have the opportunity to balance your meals and snacks. Do the best you can with what's available.

TAKE IT FROM ME...

I have known Chris Johnson professionally since the early 1980s, and have benefited greatly from him as my personal trainer both in terms of general fitness and rehabilitation for my back and knee. As a psychologist in clinical practice, I have also referred my own clients to Chris for fitness and nutrition assistance. Chris's approach has always impressed me as being balanced, holistic, and supportive of a healthy lifestyle and an optimal quality of life. His techniques are leading edge, well researched, practical, efficient, and manageable within the hectic pace of modern life. Chris is passionate about his work and demonstrates in his own life the positive results of his fitness and nutrition system.

—Alison Howie-Day, Ph.D., Licensed Psychologist

Chapter 23

MINDFUL EATING

So far, we've talked about quality carbohydrates, quality proteins, and healthy fats to satisfy the nutritional needs of our cells. *When we use our thoughts to make a plan of how, when, where, and what we will eat and then DO that plan, we are engaging in mindful eating.* But do you ever hit a bump in the road when your plans seem to disappear and you want to eat just about anything in sight, as long as it is sugary, salty, crunchy, deep-fried, and/or covered with chocolate? I've never heard anyone say they ate a whole bag of carrots in one sitting because they felt lonely. That's your clue that you may be eating to take care of some need other than feeding you cells. The purpose of this chapter is to help you become more aware of how mindless eating affects your success and to suggest some specific strategies that you could include in your action plan that will increase your mindful cating.

> Winners can tell you where they are going, what they plan to do along the way, and who will be sharing the adventure with them.
>
> —Denis Waitley

What explains overeating even after our bodies have had enough quality foods? What is this other "hunger" all about…when you can't stop thinking about ice cream, chips, cake…? In addition to hunger and the physiological triggers to overeating discussed in Chapter 10, our emotions, thoughts, habits, people, places, and events in our environment can also trigger or cue us to overeat or make unhealthy food choices. Because these cues occur so quickly, we often don't even notice what's happening until after we've eaten eight cookies, three bowls of ice cream, a bag of chips, or a sixteen-ounce steak. Ouch! This is the mindless eating cycle.

What does the mindless eating cycle look like?

1. You decide you "should" lose some weight, get stronger, more energetic.

2. You make a mental list of "forbidden" foods that you "should" permanently give up because they are "bad" for you (these are often your particular comfort foods!), and have some vague thought that you "should" exercise.

3. You get busy with life, dashing here and there. Your car has a flat tire, you have a difficult work project that is overdue, the kids are screaming, bills need to be paid, and dinner just burned on the stove. Stress builds. You feel frustrated, tired and overwhelmed.

4. You grab and q,uickly eat some (or a lot) of those comfort foods and "forget" to exercise.

5. Your light bulb goes on! You may say to yourself, "I just ate ___. I've failed once again…" and you may feel guilty, ashamed, or angry.

6. Then you may say "Well, I'm off my diet, so I might as well eat the rest of this and start again M,onday." You eat even more of the comfort food to punish yourself for eating something to comfort yourself in the first place until you feel out of control.

7. After a number of these episodes, you may say "Oh, what's the use," and give up eating healthy foods and exercising entirely. You feel discouraged and defeated.

8. You wait a period of time (days, weeks, months), realize that you still have the same problem, get your mental energy and hope up just enough to start this cycle all over again.

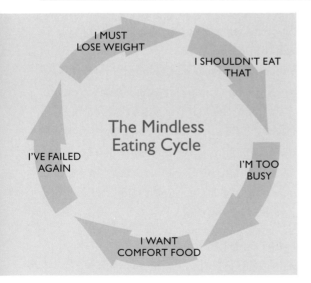

No wonder you're exhausted! This cycle creates all kinds of stress and harsh judgments of you. So how can you get yourself out of the mindless eating cycle and into the habit of mindful eating? The same way you developed new rituals for your food preparation in Chapter 16. Whether you are cued by emotions, thoughts, habits, or people, places, or events in your environment, there are strategies you can add to your action plans to overcome mindless eating.

The more mindful you are of these cues and how they affect your eating, the better prepared you are to develop new habits to achieve the success you want. If you have already made the decision to change your eating habits and you know that you engage in mindless eating that sabotages your success, a critical step to include in your action plan is to become aware of your triggers.

INCREASE YOUR AWARENESS

How are your food choices affected by your emotions, thoughts, habits, people, places, and events? What has tripped you up when you have tried to eat healthier before? What roadblocks have been in your way? A very effective strategy to add to your action plan is to use your daily food log to also *write down what was happening when you ate.* Include the time of day, how these foods got into your hands (planned or last-minute grab-and-go), what other activities you were engaged in while eating, who was present, where you were eating, and what you were thinking and feeling. Include anything that will give you clues as to why you were eating that particular food at that particular time.

The list of emotions, thoughts, habits, people, places, and events that can trigger us is endless. Each of us reacts differently to a particular cue, but here are a few examples to help you start your own awareness list.

Emotions that may contribute to mindless eating include boredom, loneliness, happiness, tiredness, anger, guilt, shame, embarrassment, deprivation, helplessness, sadness, anxiety, and fear.

Thoughts that may contribute to mindless eating include:

- Using words like "need to," "always," "never," "should," "on my diet," "off my diet," "good food," "bad food."
- "I just don't want to permanently give up so many foods I enjoy."
- "I need to keep these chips/doughnuts/pop/cookies in the house for the kids/ my partner/my dog because they are not on this 'diet' with me."
- "[fill in] will be so disappointed in me."
- "If I am thin, I am worthy."
- "If I am thin, I must be healthy."
- "I cheated on my diet."
- "I'm a failure."
- "I can't."
- "But my friends all go to lunch together and eat whatever they want, so I should be able to, too."

Some **habits** that may contribute to mindless eating include:

- Eating "comfort foods" when you feel sad, lonely, or bored.
- Eating more than 20 percent of unhealthy foods
- Eating while you watch television, surf the net, or play video games, particularly late at night. Your body "forgets" that it has eaten when you are distracted by another activity.

- Skipping meals.
- Decreasing or discontinuing your exercise.
- Becoming more reclusive, pulling away from potentially supportive relationships.
- Rewarding yourself with food when you have been "good" on your "diet."

People, places, and events in your **environment** that may contribute to mindless eating include:

- Certain people who are unsupportive or negative about your journey to become healthier, people who insist you eat "just one" of some unhealthy food that they "made just for you," or a circle of friends who only want to eat (unhealthy), drink (not water), and be merry rather than choose a healthier lifestyle.
- Certain places: lunchroom at work, restaurants, mall food courts.
- Social events: weddings, parties, holidays, sporting events.
- Advertisements in magazines, on billboards, on the radio, on the Internet, on television, on food packaging.
- The size of serving dishes used at home and in restaurants.

Do any of these sound familiar? What new cues can you add to this list from your food log notes? Your current triggers will become clearer very quickly. This strategy will give you knowledge about your specific triggers so you can build your mindful eating action plan.

BUILD YOUR MINDFUL EATING ACTION PLAN

Your action plan is the tool you use to dilute the power of your triggers. Your action plan will be very individualized and specific to you. Choose which triggers you want to start working on first and make your plan. Here are a few general strategies that you may want to include in your action plan, whether your cue is one of your emotions, thoughts, or habits or whether the cue is another person, place, or event.

Strategies

Distraction strategies can be very helpful. The purpose of adding a distraction strategy to your action plan is to change your focus from what you want to do *right now* to what you want *in the future*. When I go to the restaurant with friends, do I want to order and eat whatever everyone else is eating (right now), or do I want plan ahead to order and eat half of the plate of whole-wheat pasta with marinara sauce so I can be healthier (in the future)? Another way to change your focus is to actually change what your body is doing. This can give you enough time to *think about your action plan*. When you get an unexpected urge to eat that bag of chips, have your plan in place that you will move yourself to a different room in house; get off the couch and do an exercise tape, stretch, do yoga; call a friend and plan to get together; attend a religious service or fill your spiritual needs in some fashion; go to sleep, if you are tired; do deep-breathing exercises. *Do anything except reach into that bag of chips!*

Emotions that may help you make healthier food choices in healthier quantities include acceptance, patience, self-love, confidence, and hope. But developing strategies and action plans to manage our emotions is somewhat tricky. I don't want to suggest that you change or ignore your emotions to be successful at mindful eating. The strategy I suggest is that you *become aware of, accept, and manage your emotions.* A huge part of managing our emotions is what we believe about that emotion, what we think about when we feel that emotion, and what we do after feeling a particular emotion. *Feeling a particular emotion does NOT mean that you must think or act in a particular way!* Our feelings may just "pop up," but we can choose how we will think and act when we have that feeling. It's your action plan that focuses your thinking and action.

Thoughts are the essence of mindful eating. Our thoughts are very powerful because they drive our actions. To paraphrase Henry Ford, "Whether you believe you can or you believe you can't, you're absolutely right." One way to say "I can" is to give yourself a new script to think or say when you have thoughts that trigger you to unhealthy behavior. For example:

- Using the words "want," "sometimes," "healthier food"
- "I'm on the *Food Target* whatever I eat."
- "My kids/partner/dog can get those foods if they want them, but I don't have to bring them into the house."
- "I'm doing this healthy eating for me, because I'm worth it!"
- "I just ate a plate of french fries. Oh, there it is in the red area of the *Food Target*. That counts as some of my 20-percent choices. I'm not 'off' a diet. I'm still 'on' the *Food Target*."

Habits can be powerful tools to increase mindful eating. Add some new behaviors to your action plan that are more likely to help you make healthier food choices. If you repeat these new behaviors over and over, they will become habits. Some examples include:

- Planning meals/snacks, shopping for and preparing healthier foods more often
- Getting accurate nutritional information
- Keeping accurate food logs so you become more aware of your choices
- Eating 80 percent of your food choices from the green areas

- Learning to eat a portion of your favorite foods from the red area of the target and really enjoy every bite! Turn off the television or computer. Sit at the table and just eat. Look at it, smell it, savor the flavor in your mouth. This focused activity helps you remember that you really ate it. Then be proud of yourself that you could give yourself one of your favorite foods without feeling guilty or ashamed!
- Eating your meals at the table
- Sharing a restaurant meal with a friend or taking half of the order home for a meal the next day
- Drinking eight to ten glasses of water each day
- Taking cod liver oil daily. Cod liver oil contains vitamin D. Research shows a strong correlation between increased vitamin D and decreased depression.
- Breathing deeply several times throughout the day to relieve stress
- Getting at least six to eight hours of sleep every night
- Nurturing your spirituality in a way that fulfills you
- Eating a balance of healthy carbohydrates, proteins, and fats
- Eating every two and a half to three and a half hours
- Exercising at least thirty minutes five days a week

Environment. The tricky part about developing strategies to dilute the influence of people, places, and events is that you can't control other people, places, and events. You only have the power to choose how you respond to your environment. Behaviors that may help you make healthier food choices in relation to people, places, and events include:

- Spending time with people who genuinely support your decision to be healthier. Be aware that your circle of friends may change as your health becomes more important to you.
- Telling family and friends about your choice to live healthier and ask for their support. Be sure to tell them specifically what you want them to do to be supportive.
- Going to restaurants that have healthier menu items that you enjoy.
- Planning what you will eat at social events.
- Eating every two and a half to three and a half hours and staying well-hydrated throughout the day before you go to a special occasion so you are not ravenous. Maybe even eat just before you go if you aren't sure when the food will be available.
- Removing your trigger foods that are especially difficult for you to resist from your home.

Each action plan you develop and then do increases your mindful eating, which then creates a new healthy, balanced lifestyle cycle. This new cycle will distract you from your old thinking and behaviors and focus you on what you want, on positive thoughts and behaviors that encourage you to live a healthier lifestyle, *and* save you emotional stress and time. What a bargain!

When you practice mindful eating, your healthy, balanced lifestyle cycle looks like this:

1. You decide that you "want" to be stronger, healthier, and more energetic.
2. You make a personal mindful eating action plan that includes strategies to manage food, exercise, cues, and rewards for yourself:
   - Plan at least a few standard meals and snacks that you enjoy and that are easy to prepare. Use the principles of *On Target Living Nutrition* to eat 80 percent of your foods from the green areas of the *Food Target* and 20 percent of your foods from the outer rings, no deprivation, just eat it to get your cells healthy! Buy the food. Prepare the food.
   - Plan a specific kind of movement/exercise for a specific amount of time for five days in the upcoming week, and schedule it in your calendar.
   - Plan what you will do instead of eat when you are cued by an emotion, thought, old habit, person, place, or event.
   - Plan how you will reward yourself when you DO your action plan. Reward your healthy choices with a non-food reward that will help you continue on your journey of lifelong health. Buy a new pair of workout shoes, an MP3 player to take on your walks, or have a massage.
3. Do your mindful eating action plan and quickly eat those healthier foods that you have already prepared, or head out for your scheduled exercise, or do some deep breathing.
4. Your light bulb goes on! Yahoo for me! I can manage my busy life, eat healthy, get my workout in, and manage my (name your trigger)!
5. This is where you save time and emotional stress! Celebrate your success as your action plan becomes habit and your habit becomes ritual. Circle back to step 1 when you are ready to make more changes.

REFERENCES

The purpose of this chapter is to get you thinking about mindful eating. It is not meant to be a comprehensive discussion of the topic. There are whole books devoted to just this one aspect of unhealthy eating. If you recognize yourself in this chapter and are interested in finding more ways to create mindful eating rituals, you may find these books useful. Each of the books focuses on weight loss as the primary goal. Each contains strategies to manage how we respond to our emotions, thoughts and behaviors, people, places, and events. It's all about finding and using the tools that work best for you.

Anne Alexander, *Win the Fat War: 145 Real-life Secrets to Weight-Loss Success.* Rodale, Inc., 2000.

Phil McGraw, *The Ultimate Weight Solution: The 7 Keys to Weight Loss Freedom.* The Free Press, 2003. (The food choices are somewhat healthier, but still focus on convenience/packaged foods and omit the essential, healthy fats. Focus on the environmental strategies.)

Laurel Mellin, *The Solution: For Safe, Healthy, and Permanent Weight Loss.* Regan Books, 1997. (Excellent personal inventories and "baby-step" tools to look at the complexity of eating.)

Cathy Nonas, *Outwit Your Weight: Fat-proof Your Life with More Than 200 Tips, Tools, & Techniques to Help You Defeat Your Diet Danger Zones.* Rodale, Inc., 2002. (Excellent personal inventories and "baby-step" tools to look at the complexity of eating.)

Howard J. Rankin, *Inspired to Lose: Motivational Stories.* Step Wise Press, 2001.

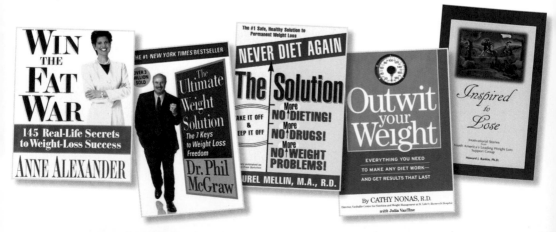

THE BOTTOM LINE

1. Accept that bumps in the road are inevitable.
2. Increase your awareness of which particular obstacles you can expect—your emotions, thoughts, habits, and people, places, and events that have tripped you up in the past.
3. Use your awareness to build your mindful eating action plan that includes strategies to manage your food, exercise, and obstacles.

TAKE IT FROM ME...

As a personal trainer I use the On Target Living principles as a tool for all of my clients and classes. I find *On Target Living Nutrition* is the most complete wellness book on the market. Instead of just telling people what they should do and eat, it arms them with the knowledge to make good choices that work for them and their family. Once you understand how to choose healthy foods and design your own exercise plan, you can follow this On Target Living program for a lifetime. As you become healthier you truly feel better, which motivates people to keep going. I find that anyone no matter where they are starting can understand Chris's program. I have used it as a tool with my clients for years and I have not found a better reference out there.

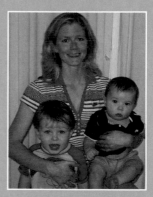

I love the book. Now I don't need any other books to supplement with my personal training with my clients or teaching classes—*On Target Living Nutrition* has it all!

Stacie Kryszak, Co-owner, The Studio: A Personal Fitness Experience

Personally, learning On Target Living changed my life. I thought I was eating fairly healthy; I was maintaining my weight and thought everything was fine. I didn't realize how much what you eat affects your overall health. I was only in my mid-twenties at the time and felt pretty healthy. I had periodontal disease, which runs in my family and I suffered from Raynaud's syndrome. Once I started eating cleaner and incorporating healthy fats, my Raynaud's disappeared and my gum disease is much better. Now I am in my thirties and have two kids and I have continued to follow Chris's way of eating. My pregnancies were healthy, my children are healthy, my weight is good, my energy is great, and I have never been healthier. The best part about On Target Living is that it gave me the knowledge to know how to make healthy choices in any situation, which made it very easy to incorporate into my daily life.

Chapter 24

HEALTHY EATING ON THE RUN

In our fast-paced lives, it can be difficult to eat in as healthy a manner as you

> Practice random acts of kindness and senseless acts of beauty.

would like, especially when you get busy or while traveling. It is easy to get out of your normal routines, and this is when you may get into trouble.

OUT-OF-TOWN TRAVEL

What do you do when you fly? Flying can truly beat you up—cramped seating, recycled air, and little to eat or drink but hydrogenated nuts, crackers, chips, cookies, soda pop, juice, alcohol, and water. You are virtually going into combat when you travel and have to be prepared! You want to feel and look your best when you arrive at your final destination. You don't have to feel like garbage every time you travel. Come prepared to feel good. I usually take a few bottles of water, balanced energy bars, fruit, and a few nuts on the plane. I never know how long the trip is going to take and don't want to depend on the airports to feed me. There is good news: many airports are now offering healthier food options.

A few years ago on a return flight from San Francisco to Michigan, I was sitting up in the bulkhead of the airplane. About three hours into the flight, I opened up some of the food that I had brought on the airplane for this five-hour flight. I had packed red peppers stuffed with tuna, nuts, and raisins. The peppers eat like an apple, are well balanced, and I like the taste. I bet you are excited about trying this crazy concoction on your next trip! Anyway, can you imagine the smell of tuna as I pulled the red peppers out of the zip-lock bag? The guy sitting next to me didn't say a thing, but ten minutes later asked, "What are you eating?" I don't think he liked the smell initially. Who would? I explained it all to him, and then he asked, "Does it taste good?"

I asked, "Would you like to try one?"

Remember, this guy has probably not eaten in five to six hours and would eat just about anything at this time! He said, "Yes, I guess so." Not the most convincing response I have ever heard, but I was not going to let this opportunity slip away. He said, "These taste better than I would have thought," and then the guy behind us who has obviously been listening to our conversation asked if he could try one!

Now I am getting really pumped. "Sure," I replied. I am sitting there watching two guys eat stuffed red peppers with tuna, what could be better? Now the red peppers stuffed with tuna may be a little extreme, but you don't have to feel like garbage when you travel. Plan ahead, come prepared, and maybe you can share a healthy snack with a new friend.

EATING OUT

Eating out is the most popular leisure activity in the United States. Almost everything we do is centered on eating. Football tailgating, graduations, weddings, retirements, holidays, entertainment, business meetings, getting together with friends—you name it, we do it with food. With the rapid growth of chain restaurants, eating out is now an everyday event for most Americans.

From a health standpoint, eating out can be a bit more challenging than eating at home. It is possible, however, to eat out and maintain healthy habits. Many restaurants have healthy choices, and the choices you make have a major impact on your health and waistline.

Here are a few tips that you can use for eating out.

Have a plan

Just like grocery shopping, eating out begins with a plan. What do you want to eat? At what type of restaurant do you want to eat? What are your options at this restaurant? How much time do you have? Take-out or sit-down? Sometimes you find yourself in situations in which you don't have much of a choice. If that is the case, focus on making the best of what is available to you.

TAKE IT FROM ME...

I have had the privilege of knowing Chris Johnson for the last six years. He has truly inspired me and made a tremendous impact on my life and on those around me. His approach to proper balance in nutrition and exercise has allowed me and all of my personal training clients to reach goals that seemed unattainable. Many lives have been changed because of his desire to help people get healthy from the inside out. Chris has earned my heartfelt appreciation and respect for all he has done and will continue to do!

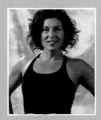

**Gay L. Byrd,
Certified
Personal Trainer,
Las Vegas, Nevada**

Make smart menu choices

Does the menu give you many options? Can you have it your way? I find most restaurants accommodating when it comes to having it your way. How is the food quality? Is the menu loaded with partially hydrogenated everything? If you are at a restaurant for the first time and are not sure of the food quality, ask if they have extra-virgin olive oil available. This does not guarantee high-quality food, but it does give you a place to start.

Let's look at an example. You have made the commitment to eating healthier. You're doing great—planning your meals and snacks—and then it hits you: the dreaded fast-food restaurant. You've been busy running around, forgotten to plan, or simply found yourself in one of those situations over which you have less control. You're hungry and need to eat. What to do? Look over the menu and examine your choices. Consider how you can eat healthy and still enjoy your meal. Do they offer a plain salad? Can you get some type of protein, like a chicken breast or some nuts, to add to your salad? Can you get oil and vinegar or a vinaigrette dressing for the salad? Think of options that will be both healthy and satisfying to you. Eating at a fast-food restaurant need not be a complete disaster of trans-fats and mega calories.

Poor fast-food choice	Better fast-food choice
large hamburger	salad of lettuce or greens
french fries	chicken breast or tuna
diet pop or milkshake	olive oil or vinaigrette dressing
	water or skim milk

Make better choices

Making better choices when eating out gets down to one thing—focus! You may want to debate me on this statement, but the next time you eat out, take a second and think about what you are focused on. I believe that what you focus on is what you will get. What are you focused on while scanning the menu? Is your focus merely on taste, or are there other factors that you want along with taste? Don't get me wrong, taste is important; I want my food to taste good too! But are you focusing on other factors that will influence your decision-making process? Are your health, your energy, and your waistline areas that you are focused on?

Every time you eat out, you will be faced with these decisions. Focus on what you want. If you know what you want, your decisions will be much easier. Should you choose the diet soda or a glass of water with lemon? The bread before lunch or dinner? The salad with bacon and ranch dressing or the salad with nuts, sprouts, extra-virgin olive oil, and balsamic vinegar? The pasta with alfredo sauce or the salmon and asparagus? The chocolate cake or a cup of sliced strawberries for dessert?

The instant gratification from food is extremely powerful, and making healthier choices can be challenging at times. As I have said throughout this book, change can be difficult, but you *can* change. Moving your attention away from just taste to other areas such as health, energy, and controlling your body weight may take time. The thought of a piece of warm bread dipped in olive oil or a slice of chocolate cake with a scoop of ice cream may sound great. We all have had these thoughts and that is okay. Food is meant to be enjoyed and shared. But can you have your cake and eat it too? Again, a big part of creating healthier lifestyle habits is what you focus on. If you truly want the warm bread or chocolate cake for dessert, then go for it and don't look back. Just be mindful of what you truly want. You may find that if you pass on the bread or cake you may feel like you have not given up anything because your focus was in a different place. You may start by focusing on drinking water with lemon instead of the diet soda pop, or eating half your entrée and taking the rest home. Eating out can be a healthy and pleasurable experience all rolled into one.

THE BOTTOM LINE

1. **Have a plan.** What do you want to eat? Where are you going to eat? Take-out or sit-down? Does the restaurant have healthy options?

2. **Scan the menu for healthy options.** Do you have many options to choose from? Can you get what you want? If you don't see what you want on the menu, ask.

3. **Focus on what you want.** Do you want good taste? Better health? High energy? A trimmer waistline? You can have it all!

4. **Ask for a take-home box.** You don't have to be captain of the clean-plate club! Ask for a box and take home a portion of your meal.

5. **Make healthier choices.** Drink water with lemon instead of a diet soda. Select extra-virgin olive oil and vinegar versus the high-fat ranch salad dressing. Choose the salmon and asparagus over the pasta with alfredo sauce. These are the choices that make the difference in what you truly want!

Chapter 25

MAKE IT YOURS

When putting together your own nutritional program, experiment with different foods and recipes. I have laid out a one-week *On Target Living Nutrition* plan. Each daily menu contains approximately 1,500 calories. Depending on your calorie needs (activity level, gender, lean muscle mass, stress, frequency of meals, and food quality), you may need to increase or decrease your quantity at each meal to alter your caloric intake. This is just a sample to demonstrate how to lay out your *On Target Living Nutrition* plan.

> All glory comes from daring to begin.
>
> —Eugene F. Ware

Personally, I am a creature of habit and eat many of the same foods every day. This makes planning, shopping, and food preparation second nature. I eat the same breakfast (oatmeal, soy milk, dried organic cherries, slivered almonds, lemon-flavored cod liver oil, and flaxseed oil) and lunch (big salad with vegetables and sprouts, chicken or fish, and extra-virgin olive oil and balsamic vinegar). I eat these two meals throughout the year. So if you find something you enjoy, don't worry about making changes every day, make it simple! There are also a food log and *Food Target* in the appendix. Make copies and use them as learning tools to plan and track your meals. Start slowly and make small changes.

Monday	
Breakfast oatmeal-on-the-run (page 227)	336 calories
Snack one cup organic yogurt with ½ cup fruit (optional: one or two teaspoons of lemon-flavored cod liver oil)	200 calories
Lunch cherry chicken salad (page 232)	264 calories
Snack flax bran muffin (page 231)	233 calories
Dinner salmon teriyaki (page 241)	216 calories
Total calories = 1,249	

Tuesday	
Breakfast CJ's special smoothie (page 231)	194 calories
Snack ½ to two-thirds cup organic low-fat cottage cheese with fruit of choice (optional: one or two teaspoons of lemon-flavored cod liver oil)	170–270 calories
Lunch CJ's big salad (page 233)	367 calories
Snack energized bar (page 230)	200 calories
Dinner buffalo or turkey meatloaf (page 239) with roasted sweet potato wedges (page 242)	337 calories
Total calories = 1,268 to 1,368	

Wednesday	
Breakfast cereal (one-half cup rolled oats or two-thirds cup dry cereal) one tablespoon slivered almonds, walnuts, or flax meal ½ cup fruit of choice ½ cup organic skim, soy, rice, oat, or almond milk	350 calories
Snack one tablespoon almonds and ½ cup of grapes	150 calories
Lunch sandwich (two slices whole-grain or sprouted bread; three ounces turkey, chicken, or tuna; tomato; romaine lettuce; mustard or canola mayonnaise) ½ cup organic low-fat cottage cheese	400 calories
Snack CJ's special smoothie (page 231)	194 calories
Dinner salmon salad (page 233)	346 calories
Total calories = 1,440	

Thursday	
Breakfast one slice whole-grain or sprouted bread two tablespoons natural peanut or almond butter apple, orange, kiwi, or a slice of melon (your choice) one hard-boiled organic free-range egg	300 calories
Snack ½ cup organic yogurt mixed with ¼ cup fruit and one tablespoon flaxseed oil or two teaspoons lemon-flavored cod liver oil	200 calories
Lunch black bean mango salad (page 232)	214 calories
Snack flax bran muffin (page 231)	233 calories
Dinner salmon patties (page 240) baked vegetables and sweet potato slices (drizzle extra-virgin olive oil and pepper, place on cookie sheet at 350°F, and bake for forty minutes) Dessert: cookies that "rock" (page 243)	452 calories
Total calories = 1,399	

Friday	
Breakfast scrambled eggs (page 229) 1 piece of fruit	300 calories
Snack CJ's special smoothie (page 231)	194 calories
Lunch cherry chicken salad (page 232)	264 calories
Snack yogurt crunch (see *On Target Living Cooking*, page 28) optional: lemon-flavored cod liver oil	201 calories
Dinner ostrich soup (page 236)	336 calories
Snack one slice toasted sprouted bread with one tablespoon organic extra-virgin coconut oil	200 calories
Total calories = 1,495	

Saturday	
Breakfast CJ's granola (page 228)	102 calories
Snack ½ cup organic yogurt with ¼ cup mixed fruit one or two teaspoons lemon-flavored cod liver oil	200 calories
Lunch leftover ostrich soup (page 236)	336 calories
Snack flax bran muffin (page 231)	233 calories
Dinner chicken and vegetable pizza (page 240)	435 calories
Snack Sliced apple with natural peanut or almond butter	150 calories
Total calories = 1,456	

Sunday	
Breakfast oatmeal pancakes (page 230)	294 calories
Snack one slice toasted sprouted bread with one tablespoon organic extra-virgin coconut oil	200 calories
Lunch grilled chicken breast black bean mango salad (page 232)	564 calories
Snack greek tomato salad (page 242)	103 calories
Dinner baked eggplant (page 241)	410 calories
Dessert apple crisp (page 245)	200 calories
Total calories = 1,771	

Chapter 26
EXERCISE:
THE FOUNTAIN OF YOUTH

When you combine daily exercise with balanced nutrition and adequate rest and recovery, the body and mind become magical. I have experienced personally and professionally the value of regular exercise and how it can transform lives. If you want to add more vitality to your life, get moving.

> Vision is the art of seeing the invisible.
>
> —Jonathon Swift

THE BIONIC WOMAN

Let me tell you about my mother, who I call the "bionic woman." At seventy-three years of age, she had suffered through an ankle fusion and replacements of both hips and a knee, all within a five-year time span. She had never been an exerciser, except for our occasional footraces in the backyard when I was a kid growing up. She actually was fairly quick! After going through post-surgical physical therapy, I nagged her about starting a regular exercise program. She resisted, arguing that she was in too much pain and didn't have the energy to devote to exercise. She also believed that exercise would increase her pain and didn't believe that it would help her.

I finally convinced her to work with a personal trainer by the name of Todd Yehl. Todd is an expert in body alignment and posture; I believe one of the best in the business. After working with Todd twice a week for six weeks, my mother felt noticeably

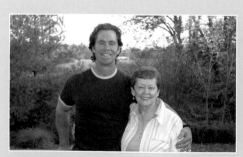

Chris and his mother, Jean

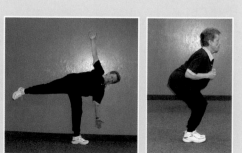

Jean enjoys the benefits of exercise

less pain and had more energy. More importantly, for the first time in many years, she had hope that her physical condition could improve. Along with improved mobility and less pain, perhaps the greatest reward has been the change in my mom's attitude. She is more active, smiles all the time, talks all the time, and has had her vitality restored! She has been exercising regularly for the past six years and works out weekly with her best friend, Dorothy. I always smile when I see Mom and Dorothy going through their exercise routines. They are both doing great! In addition, Mom is a true believer in taking her flaxseed oil, coconut oil, and cod liver oil, and drinking mineral water; she extols the benefits to anyone who will listen.

WHY DON'T WE EXERCISE?

By now, almost everyone has heard that regular exercise is good for you. Your doctor, friends, family, billboards, books, TV, radio, and health professionals all recommend regular exercise for whatever ails you. The Surgeon General reports that a sedentary lifestyle carries the same health risk as smoking, high cholesterol, diabetes, or high blood pressure. The research on the benefits of regular exercise is overwhelming. If exercise came in a pill, it would be the most prescribed medication in the world. Yet, even with all this information, research, and promotion, the United States remains a sedentary nation. Less than 25 percent of the adult U.S. population exercises on a regular basis.

Given all this information, why aren't we exercising more? With over two decades of personal training experience, and talking with friends, family, clients, physicians, and colleagues, I believe there are five major reasons why Americans are not exercising: values and beliefs, instant gratification, knowledge, time, and rituals.

Values and beliefs

We all have different values and beliefs in all aspects in our lives, and I am not here to make judgments about your values and beliefs. My goal is to get you to think about them. Values differ from beliefs. You may value success, but you may believe that to be successful you have to make over $1 million a year! You may value your health, but may believe that you must spend hours in the gym to become healthy. For a good portion of the American population, exercise is low on the priority list. For many, it is not even on the radar screen. I believe most people recognize that exercise is a good thing, but that is where their exercise wagon ends. Many feel that exercise is not for them. They may feel intimidated, uncomfortable with their body, or fear that they may fail. The list is long and, in addition, they place little value on exercise.

Exercise can be magical. Exercise can be life-changing! Exercise can improve your fitness and ability to move, decrease aches and pains, prevent injuries, improve your mood and mental clarity, decrease stress, help you sleep better, and improve your health. If you polled your friends and family members, they all would say their health is of great importance to them. They value their health, and why not? When you don't have your health, you don't have much. How valuable is your health to you? If you believe your health is important to you, what are you willing to do to maintain or improve your health? We all have to put some effort into maintaining our health. Make exercise a priority in your life. Value your health and believe you are worth it!

Instant gratification

We are a society that wants everything now. We seek instant gratification. Many of the benefits from regular exercise come later, in the form of delayed gratification. Lower cholesterol, lower blood pressure, lower body fat, improved fitness, stronger bones and muscles—you don't reap all of these benefits overnight. There have been many times when I just don't feel like exercising; I am too busy, too tired. I have all the excuses too. When I feel like this, I focus on how I will feel when I am in the middle of my exercise session and how I will feel when I am done exercising. For me, these are two powerful motivators. In the middle of my exercise routine my heart is pumping, my body is sweating, my energy has increased, and my body feels alive. After exercise my energy is high, my mind is clear, my body feels loose, and my mood is good. The feelings I get from exercising are priceless.

The most difficult time for many is just getting started. Most agree that once they begin to exercise it was not too bad and felt wonderful afterwards. In addition, there is a sense of accomplishment.

We all can learn a little from Grandma's and Grandpa's Laws. **Grandma's Law:** Eat your spinach, and then you get to have your ice cream. **Grandpa's Law:** First do your homework, and then you can go out and play.

In his book, *Emotional Intelligence,* Daniel Goleman explains a study he conducted with kids and marshmallows. The study begins by giving each kid one marshmallow. If they can delay eating the marshmallow for a certain amount of time, they are given more marshmallows. The purpose of this study was to compare instant gratification to delayed gratification and the discipline that goes with each. Dr. Goleman wanted to find out if there was a direct correlation between delayed gratification discipline and happiness. The interesting part of the study was that the same kids were monitored for over twenty years. Dr. Goleman concluded that the kids who delayed eating the marshmallow, who had the discipline to delay their gratification, became more successful, happier adults.

Don't fret if you were one of the kids who ate the marshmallow without waiting. The good news is that you can develop the skill and discipline to increase your ability to delay gratification. One of the keys for learning to delay gratification more consistently is to change your focus. Change what you place your attention on. I am going to pass on the fudge brownie with ice cream. My focus is on improving my health and having a smaller waistline.

How many times have we all said to ourselves, why did I not study enough for that final exam or why did I overeat when my goal was to lose ten pounds? In most cases we lost our focus. Remember, what you focus on is what you will attract into your life.

Knowledge

Just as with the nutritional side of the health equation, most people lack knowledge about what exercises to do, how to start, how much exercise is enough, and how to keep it going. You might want to challenge me. You might say, "Are you kidding me? Everywhere I look there are articles, books, magazines, videos, infomercials— you name it—dedicated to exercise." And as with nutrition, there's so much information that people are overwhelmed. Many people are confused about whether to do high- or low-intensity cardiovascular exercise to lose weight, which specific exercises shape or sculpt a certain body part, whether strength training is really necessary, and how much time should be devoted to what types of exercises. Now I am confused! In addition to these concerns, many people have specific questions about exercise that relate to their personal needs, such as, "If I have bad knees, Type 2 diabetes, migraine headaches, a hundred pounds to lose, pain in my shoulder, or a bad back, what exercises should I avoid? What exercises would be beneficial?"

I see evidence of the lack of knowledge and an abundance of misinformation everywhere. When visiting other health clubs, working out in hotels, listening to friends, fielding questions from participants in my seminars, I hear comments and rationales that people have constructed from myriad sources. During a recent television interview with a health and fitness expert on the subject of weight loss, the question came up about exercise and how much is necessary to lose weight. The expert recommended ninety minutes of cardiovascular exercise per day for weight loss! I almost fell over in disbelief. I thought to myself, "Is this person out of her mind?" Less than 25 percent of the American population is currently exercising, and now some expert is telling millions of viewers to exercise for ninety minutes a day to lose weight! I think many viewers were saying to themselves, "I might as well sit back on the couch and eat these cookies. There is no way I am going to exercise for ninety minutes a day." Pass the remote!

Exercise plays an important role in maintaining a healthy body weight, but it is a combination of lifestyle factors that contributes to healthy weight loss and better health. Having the right information is necessary for your success in all areas of our life. This is one reason I recommend hiring a personal trainer to help guide and educate you on developing an exercise plan that works for you. I believe everyone could benefit by hiring a personal trainer for a few sessions. You don't need to see a personal trainer three times per week. You may want to use a personal trainer weekly, or once a month for a checkup and to stay accountable. Many personal training clients say they wish they had hired a personal trainer years earlier and that it was one of the best investments they had ever made. Whether you have a bad back, pain in your shoulder, migraine headaches, want to lose weight, or want to get into the best shape of your life, there are many wonderful personal trainers to help you reach your goals. Give it a try!

At the beginning of each New Year, I see so many people desperately trying to get in better shape. "This is my year!" I believe one of the biggest mistakes people make is believing that the more time they spend on exercise the greater their results will be.

What should you look for when hiring a personal trainer? Check references. Do they have a nationally recognized personal training certification? Do they have a degree in a health-related field? How long have they been personal training? What type of clientele do they train most frequently? You are the customer; ask for what you are looking for. After reading *On Target Living Nutrition*, you will be able to ask better questions.

Time

Time is a big issue for almost everyone. I want to make this point extremely clear. *Most people don't need to spend large amounts of time to stay healthy or get into good shape.* If you are training for a marathon or the Olympics, then yes, you do have to invest large amounts of time to reach your goals. If your goal is to become healthier and get in better shape, it is important to understand that to get the most out of your exercise program, you may achieve your goals if you adjust your frequency of your exercise, the quality of the exercise you do, and the amount of time you schedule for exercise.

At the beginning of each New Year, I see so many people desperately trying to get in better shape. "This is my year!" *I believe one of the biggest mistakes people make is believing that the more time they spend on exercise the greater their results will be.* Spending more time on the treadmill or in the gym does not necessarily add up to greater results. What race are you trying to run? Is it the 100-meter sprint or the marathon? What kind of pace can you sustain for a lifetime? This is a large reason why most people slowly abandon their exercise program. It is too difficult to sustain over time. I am not saying you can't have greater focus and intensity at certain times with your exercise or nutrition program, but is this something that you can sustain? Do you want to run a sprint or a marathon? How can you incorporate exercise into your already busy life? Can you carve out five or ten minutes a day for the rest of your life to devote to exercise? I want you to get into the mindset that you need to move your body every day. Yes, every day! The human body is designed to move.

Not too long ago I was discussing this concept with a new personal training client. He was frustrated with his weight, health, and current exercise program. He said he was currently exercising for seventy-five to ninety minutes two to three times per week. His program included thirty minutes of cardiovascular excrcise followed by forty minutes of strength training and some light stretching. By the time he arrived at the gym, exercised and showered, he was spending over two hours on his exercise commitment! By listening to him I thought his exercise frequency might be the problem, so I asked again, "How often are you exercising?" He said, "two to three days per week."

Then I asked him, "How many times did you exercise last year? A hundred? A hundred and fifty? Two hundred?" This is when he spilled the beans! When he really started to analyze the frequency with which he exercised, he exercised less than thirty times last year! His life was so busy with his job and family, he just didn't have the time to devote to exercise.

So I asked him, "What kind of results do you think you would get if you exercised over 300 times a year?" Remember, he had been exercising less than once per week, and now I am asking him to exercise six times per week. I told him, "The two major changes that need to take place are to decrease your time and to increase your frequency." His new program consisted of a five- to seven-minute series of yoga and strength exercises. He did these exercises every morning before he took a shower. He also committed to at least ten minutes of walking every day and to go to the gym once each week for more strength training. This change in the quality of his workout increased the frequency to six times per week, rather than two or three, but decreased his total time commitment to about three hours, rather than six hours. An additional bonus was that he could do most of his exercise at home, to save even more time. Six months later he had lost twenty-five pounds and said he had never felt better. With his new exercise momentum, he also became more in tune with eating healthier foods. He said he never would have believed a little bit of exercise every day could really make that big of a difference. He now believes!

Developing rituals

What is a ritual? To me, a ritual is something that becomes an automatic part of you. A behavior starts as a thought, then moves into a habit, and over time may become a ritual. Rituals are similar to habits, but more powerful. A ritual is something you do on a regular basis without much thought. This is one reason it is so difficult for people to quit smoking. It has become a powerful ritual. You have a cup of coffee, you have a cigarette. You read the newspaper, you have a cigarette.

Rituals are powerful! Making my oatmeal the night before with my flax and cod liver oils has become such a ritual for me that I sometimes don't remember making it. I open up the refrigerator in the morning, and there it is! You just do it, rain or shine, without much thought or energy—like brushing your teeth, taking a shower, drinking more water, or even exercising daily.

If you are not exercising or would like to get greater results, how do you develop an exercise ritual? You must focus on what you want, why you want it and how are you going to do it. Just like your nutritional changes, take baby steps with exercise. Make it doable for you! This is one reason I have most of my clients walk for ten minutes and do a series of yoga poses for five minutes every day. It does not take much time, incorporates balance, strength, flexibility, and fitness all rolled into one, they can do it anywhere, and it makes them feel great. We can always add more to their exercise program later, but first I want them to develop some exercise rituals that will last. Imagine moving your body on a daily basis for the rest of your life. Developing healthy rituals is one of the keys to a healthier and happier you.

EXERCISE AND WEIGHT LOSS

Before I explore the specific exercise portion of this chapter, I must discuss weight loss and the mindset associated with successful weight loss. Many people I encounter have a specific goal of losing weight and believe that they will lose weight if they exercise more. Truth is, it just isn't that simple. You will burn more calories and maybe lose a few pounds by exercising more, but many people who exercise regularly are still overweight due to their poor nutritional patterns. Many folks also believe that long-duration, low-intensity cardiovascular exercise is the best method to lose weight.

Cardiovascular exercise is an important component of a balanced exercise program, but long-duration, low-intensity cardiovascular exercise is not the most efficient method for losing weight. A more successful approach to exercise takes into account the hormonal effects that occur with exercise and includes a balanced program of cardiovascular exercise, strength training, and stretching.

For many years I have competed in Natural Bodybuilding shows in the Masters Division (over age forty). This year I get to move into the Grand Master Division (over age fifty). That makes me sound as old as Lake Michigan! My exercise routine does not change a great deal prior to my contest. But nutritionally, everything tightens up. I eat more frequently, have smaller portion sizes, and take no liberties for sixteen weeks. I move from the 80/20 rule to the 95/5 rule. I cannot sustain long-term the 95/5 eating regimen. It is too strict for me. But for sixteen weeks, I can do it. I enjoy the challenge and am extremely focused. These two photos show you the changes that occurred when my exercise routine stays virtually the same, but I make significant changes in my nutrition.

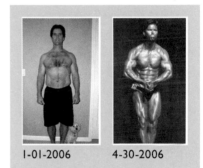

1-01-2006   4-30-2006

Proper nutrition accounts for 80 to 85 percent of successful weight loss. To get the weight loss you desire, you must begin with nutritional changes. Interestingly, while 80–85 percent of initial weight loss begins with nutrition, research shows that maintaining weight loss has to do with a combination of lifestyle factors, namely the "Big three," restful sleep, proper nutrition, and most importantly regular exercise.

POSTURE ALIGNMENT

When I was young, my grandmother always told me to "stand up straight and tall." She was so right to stress the benefits of good posture. As we age we are in a constant battle with gravity, which is trying to pull us out of ideal alignment. Daily stresses of life, sitting, standing, bending, walking, playing, and exercising challenge our ideal posture alignment. We all make some type of compromise when it comes to our posture. The challenge, and goal, is to identify our own ways of compromising and correct them, trying to improve our posture alignment.

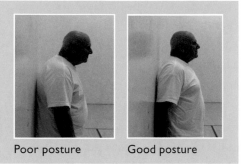

Poor posture Good posture

What is ideal posture alignment and why is it so important? Ideal posture alignment happens when the body is perfectly aligned, or in neutral position, starting with the feet and ankles, and moving up through the knees, hips, pelvis, arms, shoulders, neck, and head. The five key points for posture alignment are: the ear, shoulder, hip, knee, and ankle.

This is where exercise can be especially beneficial. We all get into repetitive movement patterns and, over time, certain muscles become shorter and stronger, while opposing muscles may become longer and weaker. This creates muscle imbalances that lead to poor posture, injury, pain, and decreased mobility. Proper exercise improves muscle imbalances and leads to better posture alignment. Having good posture is one of the key foundations to a healthier you!

A few years ago a retired, seventy-five-year-old orthodontist, Dr. Bruce Nakfoor, walked into my office complaining of back and neck pain. For years, Dr. Nakfoor had been working in a hunched-over position as an orthodontist, and over time, gravity took its toll. As part of my evaluation process, I had Dr. Nakfoor stand against the wall with his heels, glutes, and shoulders touching the wall. I think we were both surprised when his head was more than ten inches away from the wall! No wonder he was having major shoulder and back discomfort. His posture alignment needed help! So we worked on his posture, standing, sitting, and incorporated exercises he could do every day (a five-minute series of yoga/strength exercises), added some strength training, cardiovascular exercises, and good nutrition. Within three months the discomfort started to disappear, his posture improved, he lost weight, and now has started to play tennis for the first time in twenty years!

GETTING STARTED:
HOW MUCH EXERCISE IS ENOUGH?

I don't want to suggest that there is only one specific way to exercise, or that the exercises I discuss in this book are the only means to achieve the results you are seeking. My recommendations are meant to be a starting point for the new exerciser or a way to get back to basics for the experienced exerciser, who can then incorporate greater knowledge into his or her current exercise program. There are endless ways to move your body, and that's all exercise is—moving your body. Pilates, yoga, tai chi, walking, hiking, biking, using cardiovascular exercise machines, jumping rope, and swimming, skiing, surfing, strength training with free weights, rubber tubing, or machines are just a sampling of the exercises you can do on your own. Then there are the group activities like tennis, basketball, soccer, hockey, squash, racquetball, handball, playing with your kids, and exercise classes of many varieties. Your goal is to find exercises you enjoy! Get a routine, develop your exercise rituals, then over time experiment with new forms of exercise.

Personally, I do a series of foundational exercises daily that improves my strength, balance, flexibility, and posture, and they take only five to seven minutes to complete. I also walk daily. These are my everyday rituals. On top of my daily rituals I like to do twenty minutes of cardiovascular exercise, mostly on machines, and strength train for forty minutes most days. I also enjoy tennis, racquetball, swimming, skiing, and golf. Some days I need to get away from my daily routine and just play. Mixing it up keeps exercise fresh.

Remember what race are you in. Start slow, start smart. Choose ways to exercise that are fun and enjoyable for you and give you a balanced workout. Invest in yourself!

I have outlined five basic components of a balanced exercise program.

1. Dynamic warm-up: two to five minutes
2. Foundation exercises: five to seven minutes
3. Cardiovascular exercises: ten to twenty-five minutes
4. Strength training: five to forty-five minutes
5. Stretching and flexibility: three to ten minutes

TAKE IT FROM ME...

The old adage "Nothing is written in stone" certainly applies to us. As a couple in our seventies lifestyle and diet changes can occur. Under the direction of Chris Johnson and following his On Target Living principles, we have truly turned our lives around. We have been able to incorporate a more extensive exercise program, along with healthier eating habits. Our energy level and fitness have increased to the extent that we are now playing tennis, golfing, and even doing yoga exercises.

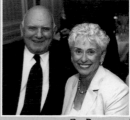

Dr. Bruce and Gloria Nakfoor

The results have been very impressive. Even our physicians have commented on the results in relationship to diabetic control and developing collateral circulation around the heart. It's been a team effort! It works! Following Chris's plan and direction, our lives have changed for the better and we are sincerely grateful.

Although each of these five components will be discussed separately, they may be integrated into one. Yoga is just one discipline or exercise that integrates all five components into one workout. Yoga combines body alignment, balance, flexibility, cardiovascular fitness, and strength together in one form of exercise. This is one reason why yoga has become more popular in the last five years in the United States.

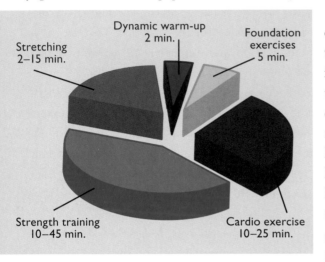

Stretching
2–15 min.

Dynamic warm-up
2 min.

Foundation
exercises
5 min.

Strength training
10–45 min.

Cardio exercise
10–25 min.

Before I go further in this exercise section I want to mention the "Rule of Training Specificity." Training specificity means that you follow a designed exercise program to fit a specific need or goal. If your goal is to become a competitive power lifter or an elite endurance athlete, you will not achieve it through yoga! However, if integrated into an athlete's exercise program, yoga can enhance that program to create better balance, flexibility, strength, and focus, and decrease the chance of injuries.

Dynamic warm-up: two to five minutes

With every form of exercise, you need time to transition your body from static or sedentary into dynamic or active. This activates the nervous, cardiovascular, and muscular systems. If you did nothing more than walk each day along with a few of these dynamic warm-up exercises, you would be ahead of the game. In my seminars I always try to get the crowd moving with a few of these exercises, and you can feel the energy in the room jump. You are probably thinking, after listening to me it has nowhere else to go but up! This is one way I get the energy back in the room, and it works every time. *Motion creates positive emotion!* I use the dynamic warm-up exercises at the beginning of all my workout sessions. The dynamic warm-up exercises cover the entire body, increase synovial fluid to help lubricate the joints, improve balance and flexibility, and are quick, taking less than five minutes. Use slow and controlled movements and gradually increase the range of motion as you warm up. If some of the movements are difficult, let pain be your guide and modify them as needed. Let the motion create positive emotion in your day!

Dynamic warm-up exercises:
- Arm swings
- Neck lateral flexion
- Neck rotation
- Round the spine
- Side bend
- Trunk twist
- Front leg swing
- Side leg swing

Foundation exercises: five to seven minutes

Foundation exercises can improve your posture, strength, balance, flexibility, and fitness all at the same time. I wanted to have a series of exercises that could improve my personal training clients' and my own personal fitness in a short amount of time. The beauty of these foundational exercises is that they don't take much time, can be done almost anywhere with no equipment requirements, and, most of all, they work.

I have all of my personal training clients using the foundation exercises in some manner every day. You may to

> Practice does not make perfect. Only perfect practice makes perfect.
>
> —Vince Lombardi

choose to modify each movement or add or delete any of the exercises to fit your current needs. You may choose to do foundation exercises before you play golf, tennis, basketball, bike, walk, jog or run, lift weights or just as your main source of exercise for that day. Hold each exercise for five to twenty seconds, and focus on the proper technique for each movement.

1. Standing or seated posture
2. Squat
3. Straight leg lunge—warrior 3—half moon
4. Warrior 1 and 2—reverse warrior—extended angle
5. Standing spread eagle
6. Dancer
7. T-extensions
8. Half moon (against the wall)
9. Standing up-and-down dog

See Appendix B, page 251 for specific information.

Cardiovascular exercise: fifteen to thirty minutes

When most people think of cardiovascular exercise, they think of walking, jogging, biking, swimming, cross-country skiing—virtually any exercise that is rhythmic in nature. Cardiovascular exercise places demands on the heart, lungs, and muscles. There are many benefits including stress reduction, improved pH balance, mood elevation, increased cardiovascular efficiency, decreased blood pressure, improved blood glucose, lipids, weight control, and, most of all, it makes you feel good!

Cardiovascular exercise can be either aerobic or anaerobic or somewhere in between, depending on the intensity level of the exercise. *Aerobic exercise* occurs when the demand of exercise *meets* the supply of oxygen. *Anaerobic exercise* occurs when the demand of exercise *exceeds* the supply of oxygen.

It is important to understand the difference between aerobic and anaerobic exercise and how the intensity of your exercise program can affect certain hormones and, more importantly, help you get the results you desire. Your "fountain of youth" hormones, testosterone (produced by both men and women), and human growth hormone, are stimulated by higher-intensity anaerobic exercise. These two hormones help the body become leaner, stronger, and more youthful.

Quality versus quantity

When educating my personal training clients about cardiovascular exercise, I explain that as their cardiovascular fitness levels start to improve, the goal is not to increase the length of time dedicated to cardiovascular exercise, but to slowly increase the intensity level, or difficulty, of that exercise.

I believe many people look at cardiovascular exercise as a way to burn calories and lose weight, assuming more time is better. This is not necessarily true. *If your goal is weight loss, it is far more effective and more efficient to limit the time spent on cardiovascular exercise to twenty to thirty minutes, but raise the intensity.* The higher intensity and corresponding stimulation of testosterone and human growth hormone will have a greater impact on weight loss than tracking the number of calories burned.

It sounds simple. To lose weight using cardiovascular exercise, increase the intensity and go like mad! But hold on. There are a few other things you must understand about high-intensity cardiovascular exercise. First, high-intensity exercise day in and day out is tough, and can turn you off to exercise altogether. Personally, I work hard during the cardiovascular section of my workout, but in most cases I am not torturing myself. Second, it is more difficult to maintain good posture with higher-intensity cardiovascular exercise. Pay attention to your posture the next time you go for a walk, jog, ride your bike, or get on your favorite cardiovascular exercise machine. Maintaining good posture will increase the difficulty of each exercise. Poor postural alignment may lead to orthopedic problems and injuries.

The biggest reason that you should not spend excessive time doing cardiovascular exercise is the hormonal changes that begin to occur. Testosterone and growth hormone levels begin to drop after twenty-five to thirty minutes of cardiovascular exercise. These are the hormones that stimulate muscle growth and make the body leaner. *Human growth hormone is the most powerful fat-burning hormone in the body.* So it does not make much sense to exercise longer if one of your goals is weight loss. On the other hand, as the length of your cardiovascular session increases, cortisol, your "stress" hormone, begins to rise. Excessive levels of cortisol can cause bone loss, muscle wasting, thinning skin, hypertension, poor wound healing, impaired immune function, and weight gain. No other hormone in the human body ages you faster than cortisol!

If you are an endurance athlete, you need to put in more time. This is the rule of training specificity. If you enjoy going for a leisurely long walk or bike ride, do it and enjoy all the wonderful benefits that follow. But if your goal is to improve your fitness, health, and weight control, start adding short bouts of higher-intensity effort throughout your cardiovascular exercise program as you become more efficient with your exercise time. The benefits of cardiovascular exercise do not increase by adding more time to your program; fifteen to thirty minutes of moderate- to high-intensity cardiovascular exercise are all that's needed!

Clients tell me that one of the main barriers to regular exercise is a lack of time. Time is precious. Don't waste it with unnecessary cardiovascular exercise. Unless your goal is to participate in endurance activities such as long-distance marathon running or triathlons, stick with shorter-duration, moderate- to higher-intensity cardiovascular exercise. Start slowly and progress gradually to allow your body time to adapt to the demands of exercise.

Cardiovascular exercise outline

Modality: It's what you do. Find an exercise you enjoy and add variety to your workouts. Walking, biking, swimming, running, hiking, snowshoeing, cross-country skiing, group fitness classes, and using cardiovascular machines are just a few of the cardiovascular exercises that many people enjoy.

Frequency: It's how often you do it. Try to develop exercise patterns that fit your available time and schedule. Exercise two to seven times a week.

Duration: It's how long you do it. Even ten minutes of cardiovascular exercise can have many benefits. Ideally, try to get fifteen to thirty minutes and pay attention to posture and intensity level.

Intensity: It's how hard you work. "Intensity" means the level of difficulty in sustaining the exercise. If the exercise is so hard that you can last only a few minutes before you have to stop, your intensity level is too high. If your intensity level is too low, your body will make only minimal adaptations and you will get fewer benefits from the exercise session.

Four methods to monitor exercise intensity

Visual: Watch your body language and postural alignment. If the intensity is too high, the body begins to make compensations, leading to a breakdown in postural alignment.

Talk test: As exercise intensity increases, it becomes more difficult to talk. The body is switching energy systems from aerobic to anaerobic metabolism. If you can easily carry on a conversation, your intensity may be too low. If you can say only a few words without stopping to catch your breath, your intensity is too high. Find the balance that is specific to your goals.

Perceived exertion: Assess your level of exertion on a one-to-ten scale, with one to two being easy, four to six moderate, and eight to ten extremely difficult.

Heart rate: Traditionally, this is the gold standard for monitoring exercise intensity. As exercise intensity increases, heart rate increases. Use the following formula to find a target heart rate zone. Take 220 minus your age and multiply this number by how hard you want to exercise. A beginning level, or lower intensity level, would be 50 to 60 percent. The maximum or highest-intensity level is 80 to 90 percent. Let's figure out a heart rate zone to fit a forty-year-old person's fitness level.

Intensity	Age	Intensity	Heart rate
Easy:	220 – 40 (age) =	180 × 50% =	90 bpm (beats per minute)
Moderate:	220 – 40 (age) =	180 × 60–70% =	108–126 bpm
High:	220 – 40 (age) =	180 × 80–90% =	144–162 bpm

If you are just getting started with exercise, start slowly and keep your heart rate around 90 to 107 beats per minute (bpm). For a moderate exerciser, 108 to 126 bpm would be the goal. For the advanced exerciser or when doing interval training, 144 to 162 bpm is the target. These are just guidelines. Monitor your heart rate further with the talk test and by assessing your perceived exertion to see how your heart rate measures up.

The challenge of monitoring your heart rate is that it uses age as a predictor of fitness level, which can be inaccurate. If you are on any medications, especially cardiac medications, the medication may affect heart rate levels. It's important to use all the methods to monitor the intensity level of your exercise.

It is always a good idea to consult with your doctor or exercise professional before beginning any exercise program. Remember to start slow and let your body slowly acclimate to your exercise program.

Strength training: five to forty-five minutes

If there is one form of exercise that can turn back the hands of time, it is strength training. More and more, people reap its benefits. Even people in their eighties and nineties can improve their strength, mobility, and bone density with strength training. I have seen the benefits of strength training with many of my personal training clients who have trained with me for many years. The benefits of strength training include increased strength, increased bone density, improved mobility and functionality, improved posture, better balance, fewer injuries, improved athletic performance, reduced stress, increased self-esteem, increased metabolism, and weight control.

Strength training is exercise that uses resistance to place demands on the nervous system, hormones, bones, and muscles. Strength training is generally done with a short burst (ten to thirty seconds) of the strength training phase, followed by a recovery phase. The rest or recovery phase can last ten seconds to four minutes, depending on your goals.

With the right intensity, strength training taxes the anaerobic system and stimulates testosterone and human growth hormone. Women, don't be afraid that you will bulk up with strength training. Men have a great deal more testosterone than women do. It takes a tremendous amount of effort, good nutrition, and the right parents to get larger muscles. I have been trying to build bigger muscles for years, and it is difficult to do!

Recently at one of my seminars I was asked the question, "How long have you been strength training?" I have been strength training for over thirty-five years! When I was younger, my main goal was to build larger muscles and enhance my athletic performance. I will turn fifty this year, and am still trying to build bigger muscles. But strength training does so much more than build larger muscles! Strength training improves posture and balance, prevents injuries, reduces stress, improves mobility, increases confidence, increases bone density, improves athletic performance, and most of all improves the way you feel. Strength training increases one's *vitality!* After I strength train, my mind is clear, my mood is great, and I feel energized.

Strength training can be done with a variety of equipment. Use your own body weight, free weights, rubber tubing, or strength training machines, to name a few. As you begin your strength training program, focus on the following guidelines:

1. **Good posture:** Before the start of each exercise get into good posture and maintain this posture alignment throughout the entire exercise. When you're postural alignment begins to break down, stop the exercise.

2. **Focus:** Concentrate on the exercise you are performing. How is your posture? What muscles are you trying to engage? Are you making a connection between the brain and the muscles, using the body's neuromuscular system?

3. **Technique:** Are you doing the exercise correctly? This is a big one. Doing an exercise correctly is everything! The right strength training technique does matter. I see so many people just walk into the strength training room, jump on a piece of equipment or pick up free weights and go at it, with no idea how to do the exercise correctly. The exercises in this book are just a sample of what's out there. Hiring a personal trainer for a few sessions to learn proper exercise technique is money well spent. Invest in yourself!

4. **Proper progressions:** There's more to strength training than repetitions, sets, and resistance. As your body adapts to your strength training program, start making a few small changes in your program so your body stays challenged and continues to make adaptations. These seven areas of progressions include number of exercises, sets, repetitions, resistance, rest and recovery, speed of movement, and stability and balance.

   Number of exercises: The big question is how many exercises to do. If you are just beginning, work the entire body by doing four to six exercises. As you advance, add a few more exercises or divide your routine into splits (upper body on the first day, lower body on the second day).

   Sets: Start with one set of each exercise. As you advance, move to two to four sets per exercise.

   Repetitions: Within each set, do from six to twelve repetitions, or "reps." Use reps as a guideline to measure your intensity and progress. More important than the number of reps is your technique and maintaining proper posture throughout each exercise movement. If your posture breaks down, regardless of your desired rep range, stop the exercise. Losing proper posture is how people get injured or develop muscle imbalances and poor movement patterns.

Resistance: Resistance is the load used in any given set or rep. Choosing the correct resistance can be a bit challenging at first. Your goal with every exercise is to create and maintain good posture alignment and then add resistance to challenge the muscular system. I tell my clients, "Listen to your body, maintain perfect form, and don't get caught up in just pushing weight."

Rest and recovery: The more intensity, reps, and resistance in each exercise set, the more recovery time will be necessary between sets. If your goal is to max out during with a specific amount of resistance, you will need a longer recovery time between sets (one to three minutes). Rarely do I lift my maximal amount of weight in a specific exercise, but if this is one of my goals then I will need much more recovery time between sets. If your goal is to integrate many exercises with a moderate amount of resistance, you will have shorter recovery times (ten to forty-five seconds) between sets.

Speed of movement: Speed of movement is an important tool to help monitor the intensity of each exercise. Begin with a two-second count in both phases of the strength movement, making the total time for each rep four seconds. I will use a pushup as an example. Take approximately two seconds to lower your chest to the floor, and two seconds to come up. Experiment with the speed of your strength movements; it is a great way to keep your training fresh.

Stability and balance: As you improve and become fit, start challenging your stability and balance. When you are beginning, it is much easier to strength train while you are stable (sitting at a chest press machine as opposed to doing a pushup while your toes are up on a Swissball or step).

5. **Breathing:** Do not hold your breath when strength training. Ideally, exhale during the exertional phase and inhale during the recovery phase of the strength movement. Most importantly, try to keep your breathing regular.

Stretching/flexibility: three to ten minutes

There are many benefits of stretching the muscles of the body, from decreasing stress to improving muscle imbalances. Stretching exercises should be performed only after the body is warmed up. You would not want to stretch a rubber band after it was in the freezer, and the same is true with your muscles and connective tissue. So spend some time getting your core temperature up before you begin to stretch. This is one reason why dynamic exercises are done at the beginning of your workout and stretching and flexibility are performed at the end of a workout or after the body is warmed up. There are hundreds of different stretching exercises from which to choose. I have chosen a few basic stretches that cover the entire body. Don't neglect the stretching portion of your exercise program. Start with just a few stretches and build the habit of stretching. I have most of my personal training clients do at least the standing up-and-down dog stretch. Both are easy to perform and stretch many areas of the body. Focus on proper alignment and deep, slow breathing. Stretching exercises may be done daily. A few general rules to follow:

1. Hold each stretch for ten to sixty seconds.
2. Maintain ideal posture throughout all stretches.
3. Do not stretch to a point of pain or discomfort.

Stretches:
1. Cat and dog
2. Modified downward dog
3. Modified upward dog
4. Downward dog
5. Upward dog
6. Warrior 1 and 2, extended angle, reverse warrior, spread eagle
7. Warrior 3
8. Dancer
9. Half moon against the wall
10. Kneeling hip flexor
11. Modified camel/camel
12. Advanced hamstring
13. Child's pose
14. Frog stretch
15. Big three tubing
16. Supine hip stretch
17. Piriformis 1 and 2

EQUIPMENT NEEDS

Very little equipment is needed for the dynamic warm-up, foundations, and cardiovascular exercises that I recommend. For strength training start by using your own body weight, such as a squat, straight-leg yoga lunge, or modified pushup. Using exercise rubber tubing is also an easy way to start. Exercise tubing comes in many colors, each representing different levels of resistance. I use the exercise tubing in my own training and also with most of my personal training clients. I highly recommend **Gym on the Go** to help guide you through your tubing workout. The Gym on the Go product contains exercise tubing and an easy-to-follow video and guide. For information about Gym on the Go, visit www.gymonthego.com.

It is also a good idea to purchase a few dumbbells. A good starter set includes three-, five-, eight-, ten-, twelve-, fifteen-, and twenty-pound dumbbells.

I also recommend purchasing a Swissball. These come in different sizes, 55 cm for people five feet eight or under and 65 cm for those five feet nine or taller. Finally, I recommend purchasing an adjustable bench and a yoga mat for floor and stretching exercises. The ball, bench, and mat can be purchased at your local sporting goods or fitness equipment store or online.

SAMPLE EXERCISE PROGRAMS

I have designed a few sample exercise routines for the beginner, intermediate, and advanced exerciser. The goal with all exercises is to challenge the body while maintaining ideal posture and good technique throughout each exercise. Start slowly and listen to your body. See Appendix B, page 281.

FREQUENTLY ASKED EXERCISE QUESTIONS

1. **If exercise is so good for us, then why don't more people do it?**
   For many, it is the time element. People feel they just don't have time to exercise. In reality, you cannot afford *not* to exercise. Plan exercise into your schedule and make it a priority. Also, exercise needs to be fun and enjoyable. Experiment with your exercise program and try to include activities you enjoy.

2. **How much exercise is enough?**
   This depends on your personal goals. If you want to achieve a very high fitness level, then the time needed for exercise will be greater than someone who wants to develop basic conditioning. One of the magical things about the human body is that it gets better with use. You do not have to spend a lot of time to keep your body in good condition. Small doses of exercise on a consistent basis are very beneficial. Developing consistent exercise habits will give you the greatest long-term benefits. Start slowly with your program and begin to develop good exercise patterns.

3. **Do I need to buy special exercise machines and equipment to get a good workout?**

   Not at all. The only exercise tool that is necessary is your own body. You may want to supplement your program with other equipment, but it is not necessary.

4. **Is it expensive to start an exercise program?**

   No. If you would like to get started in your own home, you can start without spending any money. Or you may elect to outfit your home with some exercise equipment at a very low cost.

5. **How should I breathe when exercising?**

   Never hold your breath during exercise. Holding your breath during exercise may increase your blood pressure. When strength training, exhale during *exertion.*

6. **Does exercise have to be painful to get results?**

   Many times you may experience some discomfort when exercising. For instance, you may be out of breath or feel some burning in your muscles. If you are experiencing true pain, your body is signaling you to slow down or to stop. Exercise should not be painful to perform. It may become difficult at times, but should never be painful.

7. **Can exercise be fun and enjoyable?**

   Fitness professionals agree that for people to stay with any exercise program, it *must* be fun and enjoyable. Use exercises you enjoy, not just exercises you think are good for you.

8. **When is the best time to exercise?**

   The core body temperature for most people reaches its peak during the late afternoon and early evening. This is the easiest time for the body to perform at its best. Many people, however, exercise when it fits their schedule. Depending on your goals, schedule time for your exercise program that fits best for you and stick with it. Plan your exercise time.

9. **Should I eat before I exercise?**

   If you are exercising first thing in the morning you may want to eat after you exercise. A small balanced snack or meal approximately 1½ hours prior to and after exercise is recommended. If you find you don't have much energy to exercise, focus on eating better, good sleep habits, and balance in your current lifestyle.

10. **What causes muscle soreness and what should I do about it?**

Muscle soreness is caused by micro-tears in the muscle. Most muscle soreness reaches its peak forty-eight hours after exercise (commonly referred to as *delayed onset muscle soreness*). Activity that overloads muscle in ways it is not accustomed to can cause muscle soreness.

11. **Is muscle soreness good?**

It depends on how severe the soreness is. If you are so sore you can hardly walk, this is an indication that your activity level was too severe, and that your progression into the activity was too quick. A small amount of muscle soreness can be beneficial. This slight soreness is an indication that your activity is progressing in the right direction. You are achieving a training effect.

Active rest, such as walking, stretching, easy swimming, sauna, hot tub, or massage, is an excellent way to help recover from muscle soreness. Remember to enjoy your fitness program and make gradual yet continuous improvements.

12. **How important are rest and recovery?**

Adequate rest and recovery times are essential for good, long-term health and fitness. Give each muscle group a day off between workouts to allow the muscle fibers to rebuild. To perform at your optimum level, you need adequate sleep, relaxation time, active rest, and good nutrition. If you do not allow for adequate rest and recovery, your potential for injury and burnout increases.

13. **Should I exercise every day?**

Moving the body on a regular basis is an important ingredient in keeping the body healthy. Strength training can put great demands on the body. Adequate recovery between strength-training sessions is important for achieving the greatest benefits. Get one to two days of rest between body parts if you are splitting your training sessions into specific body parts. For example, if you are training the chest muscles on Monday, you can train your back muscles on Tuesday. Cardiovascular and flexibility training can be done on a daily basis. Start slowly, listen to your body, and take days off as needed.

EXERCISE CONSIDERATIONS

1. You may wish to consult your physician or exercise professional before you begin your exercise program. I highly recommend hiring a qualified personal trainer for three to five sessions to get you started on the right track.
2. Make sure you are well-hydrated before, during, and after exercise.
3. Exercise greatly increases body temperature. Be careful when exercising in a warm environment.
4. Wear comfortable, breathable clothing when exercising. Buy a good pair of shoes to wear during exercise.

THE BOTTOM LINE

1. Fewer than 25 percent of the American population exercises on a regular basis. I believe there are five major reasons why many people don't exercise: values and beliefs, instant gratification, time, knowledge, and rituals.
2. Motion creates positive emotion!
3. Find exercises you enjoy.
4. Move you body every day.
5. Schedule time to exercise.

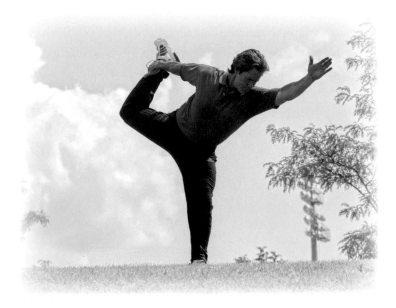

Chapter 27
STARTING AT ZERO

At this point in this book your brain may be hurting, and you may be thinking that this is getting pretty overwhelming! You may not be eating as healthy as you would like, your energy is low, your stress is high, and you seldom move your body. You want to be healthier and have more energy. You look at the *Food Target* and see that most of what you are eating is in the red area. You know you need to take that first step but are not sure where to start. Sometimes getting started is the most difficult part of the journey.

> When we have done our best, we should wait the result in peace.

A few years back while doing a seminar in Michigan for a large group of dental hygienists, one of my lifelong friends, Wayne Jackson, was helping me sell books in the back of the room. Wayne is fifty-five years old, is in great shape, and is a wheat grass disciple. I told him a few years ago that wheat grass helps retard grey hair and he has been hooked ever since! Wayne's energy and passion for life are contagious, and I always enjoy spending time with him. Wayne is also good for business; seldom does anyone get out of the room without buying a book or two. On this day Wayne said to me, "You cannot believe how many people came up to me after your seminar, highly motivated to make some changes, but felt like they were starting at zero. Most of what they had been eating was on the outside of the *Food Target*." He added, "In the future you need to talk more about starting at zero and how to take that first step. People need to know they have hope that small changes can truly make a difference over time."

TAKE IT FROM ME...

I have always believed that physical fitness is the key to maintaining a balanced lifestyle. Fifteen years ago I became a certified personal trainer and it was at this time that I became familiar with Chris Johnson's integrative approach to On Target Living. On Target Living is the perfect balance of how to make everyday rest, food, and exercise choices that will maximize your sense of well-being while ensuring your overall health and fitness. We all start from zero and creating healthy lifestyle habits can lead to greater health and happiness.

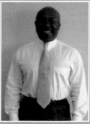

Wayne Jackson

I believe that I owe my overall sports performance, improved physical fitness, and greater health and well-being to incorporating the On Target Living principles into my daily life. CJ, thanks for the opportunity to comment and also for being a solid trusting friend for more than thirty years.

Recently I used the starting-at-zero concepts with my dad. My dad and I have a great relationship. We all want the best for our parents and in the last few years, I, along with my sister and brother, have been concerned with Dad's health. Dad's health and fitness level have slowly deteriorated over the years. He has never been overweight and has always "looked" to be in good shape. Unfortunately, taking care of his health has never been high on his priority or values list, regardless of strong encouragement from his kids. I have always told Dad, "You don't know how good you could feel. If you just did a little bit each day, you would be amazed how your health and energy could improve."

While returning from a golf trip with my dad, the conversation came up surrounding health and fitness and his need to get in better shape. His fitness level was quickly deteriorating and he was becoming more concerned about his shortness of breath. He was even having trouble getting the golf ball out of the hole due to his hip and leg discomfort. Dad has never been interested in learning the ins and outs of nutrition or fitness, so I asked him, "What if you did just one or two things a day that would help improve your health and make you feel better?" I asked him if he would be interested in a simple plan that was doable for him. My dad was starting at zero and needed to take that first step. I said to Dad, "Each day I want you to drink two or three bottles of water, walk for ten minutes, and eat one or two carbohydrates, one or two proteins, and one or two fats coming from the inner two circles (green areas) of the *Food Target*. You don't have to eat all of your foods from the green areas, just one or two from each of the three categories. No calculations, no measuring, just developing daily habits of drinking water, walking, and eating a few foods from the inner circles of the *Food Target*."

Then he asked, "Is this all I have to do? Will this really make a difference?"

I said, "When was the last time you drank two bottles of water or went for a ten-minute walk? If you follow these basic practices every day, you will be amazed how good you can feel."

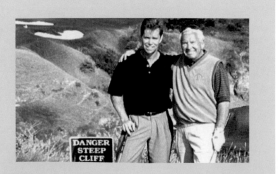

Here is my dad's starting-at-zero plan:
- Drink two or three bottles of water per day.
- Walk for ten minutes per day.
- Eat one or two carbohydrates, proteins, and fats from the inner two circles (green areas) of the *Food Target*.

If you feel that you are starting at zero, don't worry. Use the *Food Target* to help you make your changes. If most of what you are currently eating is on the outer ring of the *Food Target*, just try to move slowly towards the center. If you are currently eating sugared cereal for breakfast, you don't have to switch to steel-cut oats tomorrow.

Some transitions in the *Food Target* are easier than others. For example, you may currently use peanut butter made with partially hydrogenated oils (trans-fats), which is located in the outer ring (red area) of the *Food Target*. Moving from unhealthy peanut butter to natural peanut butter (in the gold area of the *Food Target*) is an easy switch to make. The price is the same, it's easy to find, and it tastes good. One complaint I hear about natural peanut butter is that it gets hard after you put it in the refrigerator. To keep your natural peanut butter soft and creamy, stir it up, turn it upside down, and place it in the refrigerator. No more stiff peanut butter for you!

Use the *Food Target* as a tool to help guide your choices. Your goal is to make small changes that you can live with and develop healthier habits over time. It is these small changes that make a big difference over time.

I have a sample starting-at-zero plan that can give you a few ideas to get started. You don't have to do everything on day one. Pick just one or two areas you want to improve on, make it simple, and just do it!

Regular exercise improves your health, energy, mood…the list is long.

Remember when starting at zero, begin slowly and build on your successes. Your goal is to build healthy rituals into your day!

TAKE IT FROM ME...

Meeting Chris Johnson five years ago has changed my life. Without even realizing it, Chris began motivating me to follow my dream of teaching ways to live a healthy lifestyle. I have watched and listened as Chris takes his audience through the journey of On Target Living. His motivation makes you want to change your lifestyle, but it's his passion that makes you believe you can do it. *On Target Living Nutrition* is a simple plan that has changed so many lives. I have gone from being a participant in this healthy lifestyle to teaching it daily. In my journey of following Chris's footsteps I have seen firsthand what *On Target Living Nutrition,* along with exercise, can do: weight loss, increased energy, improved blood chemistry, improved mental health, and much more. It takes commitment, but the rewards are overwhelming. I cannot think of a better motivator, teacher, and friend to have on this journey than Chris Johnson.

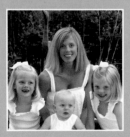

Kelley Foltz, Certified Personal Trainer

Enjoy the journey!

Sample starting-at-zero plan

1. **Water:** Start with thirty to fifty ounces of water per day (spring water, artesian water, mineral water). The human body is 70 percent water, and staying properly hydrated is extremely important for health and performance.

2. **Carbohydrates:** Move closer to the center of the food target.
   Fruits: Fruits are high in many essential vitamins, minerals, antioxidants, and fiber; most fruits are alkaline and give us energy. Eat one or two fruits per day (oranges, apples, berries).
   Vegetables: Vegetables are high in many essential vitamins, minerals, antioxidants; most vegetables are alkaline and give us energy. Eat one to three vegetables per day (broccoli, asparagus, leafy greens).
   Whole Grains: Whole grains are loaded with fiber, vitamins, and minerals and give us energy. Eat one or two whole grains per day (oatmeal, rye, wheat, millet).

3. **Proteins:** Move closer to the center of the food target. High-quality proteins help stabilize blood glucose, boost the immune system, and are used as building blocks in the body. Eat two or three servings of high-quality proteins (nuts, seeds, whole grains, vegetables, dairy products, fish, eggs, meats).

4. **Fats:** Move closer to the center of the food target. Healthy fats improve cellular health, hormonal balance, and satiety, and give us energy. Eat two or three tablespoons of healthy fats per day (almonds, walnuts, extra-virgin olive oil, and flax meal or flaxseed oil, cod liver oil).

5. **Frequency:** Eat three to five small meals per day. Eating small meals frequently improves energy, increases metabolism, stabilizes blood glucose, and decreases fat-storing lipase enzymes.

6. **Rest/Recovery:** Do deep breathing exercises for thirty seconds twice a day. Set up patterns for a good night's sleep (seven to eight hours per night).

7. **Exercises:**
   Pay attention to your *posture.*
   Walk for ten minutes per day.
   Foundational exercises: five minutes per day.

Chapter 28

TAKING IT TO THE NEXT LEVEL

Now that you have had a glimpse of the starting-at-zero plan, what do you do if you want to dial it up a bit? Where do you want to go with your health and fitness needs, and how much do you want to invest? Maybe you have already made many wonderful changes but now are ready for more. Maybe you want to drop a few more pounds, wean your-

> ## Change starts when someone sees the next step.
>
> —William Drayton

self off one of your medications, become fit, climb a mountain, or have more vitality in your life. How do you take it to the next level?

Not long ago, I began working with a female triathlete by the name of Kate DiMeo. Kate's goal was to lose a little body fat, increase her energy, stay healthy, and elevate her performance in competition. She was fit and trim, but she felt she could be better. We went over her current nutritional program and found she was eating too many empty, low-quality foods, foods on the outer rings of the *Food Target*. She was also skipping meals as a way to keep her calories down and was not getting a good variety or a good balance in her diet. After that session, she went right out and changed her nutritional plan overnight! She improved the quality of her food and drink choices, ate every three hours, added a variety of healthy fats, and started taking wheat grass along with a large salad with vegetables for lunch. She also added a daily regimen of foundational exercises to improve her alignment, strength, flexibility, and balance. At the end of the first week, I asked her to send me a food log to monitor her progress.

Kate's Food Log

7:30 a.m.:	Frozen wheat grass cube in lemon sparkling water
8:00 a.m.:	½ cup dry rolled oats, ½ cup plain almond milk, one tablespoon flaxseed oil, two teaspoons cod liver oil, 1 banana
11:00 a.m.:	Chicken breast and yam
2:00 p.m.:	Salad with broccoli slaw, sprouts, carrots, broccoli, cauliflower, beets, chicken, hummus, extra-virgin olive oil, and balsamic vinegar
6:00 p.m.:	Smoothie with one scoop of soy-based protein powder, ½ cup frozen strawberries, ½ cup organic plain yogurt, and twelve ounces water
9:00 p.m.:	One piece of toasted organic sprouted bread with 1 tablespoon organic extra-virgin coconut oil and 1 tablespoon organic strawberry jam
9:30 p.m.:	Twelve ounces mineral water with a shot of organic pomegranate juice, two evening primrose capsules

I don't want her food log to scare you. Most people will normally implement a few changes, but rarely do they do almost everything that we discussed in our consultation. If you want to take your current program up a notch, I have put together a sample plan that you may want to adapt.

TAKING-IT-TO-THE-NEXT-LEVEL PLAN

1. **Water:**
   - Drink half your body weight in ounces of water per day.
   - Choose from spring water, artesian water, ionized water, or well water.
   - Drink twelve to sixteen ounces of mineral water per day.
   - The human body is 70 percent water, and staying properly hydrated is essential for good health and performance.

2. **Carbohydrates:** Move to the inner two circles (green areas) of the *Food Target.*
   - *Fruits:* two per day (berries, oranges, apples)
   - *Vegetables:* two to five per day (leafy greens, broccoli, asparagus)
   - *Whole grains:* one or two per day (oatmeal, amaranth, millet, rye)
   - *Legumes:* one or two per day (lentils, beans)
   - *Starchy carbohydrates:* one or two per day (yams, purple potatoes, whole-grain rice)
   - Nutrient-dense carbohydrates contain essential vitamins, minerals, fiber, and improve mood and give us energy.

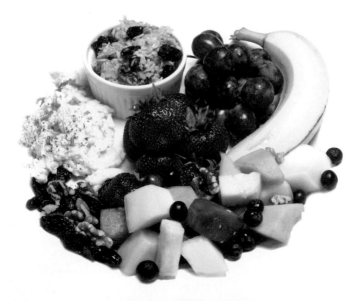

3. **Proteins:** Move to the inner two circles (green areas) of the *Food Target*.
   - Plant-based proteins such as nuts, seeds, whole grains, and vegetables should make up a great deal of your protein requirements.
   - Use only organic animal sources of protein whenever possible.
   - Consume half of your body weight in grams of protein per day.
   - High-quality proteins help stabilize blood sugar, boost the immune system, and act as building blocks in the body.

4. **Fats:** Move to the inner two circles (green areas) of the *Food Target*.
   - *Trans-fats.* Avoid all trans-fats. If a product lists partially hydrogenated oils in its ingredient list, it contains trans-fats.
   - *Saturated fats:* Organic extra-virgin coconut oil is a wonderful-tasting and healthy fat, one tablespoon per day. Great for high temperature heat and baking. Improves digestion, nutrient absorption, acid reflux, thyroid function, skin, immune system, and weight loss.
   - *Monounsaturated fats:* Extra-virgin olive oil, almonds, almond oil, macadamia nut oil, avocados. One or two tablespoons per day. Great for cooking, improves HDL and LDL cholesterol, blood pressure, and hormonal balance.
   - *Omega-3 essential fatty acids:* Flax meal, flaxseed oil, walnuts, leafy greens, cod liver oil, wild cold-water fish. One or two tablespoons per day. Improves cellular health, hormonal balance, brain function, cholesterol, and energy, and decreases inflammation.
   - *Omega-6 essential fatty acids:* Evening primrose oil, borage oil, pumpkin seeds/oil, sesame seeds/oil, sunflower seeds/oil. One or two tablespoons per day. Improves cellular health, hormonal balance, and absorption of healthy fats.
   - Healthy fats are the body's healing nutrients. Getting a variety of healthy fats is critical for the body performing at its best.

5. **Miscellaneous foods, beverages, and supplements:** Health enhancing.
   - *Wheat grass:* One of nature's true super foods. Wheat grass contains over ninety-two minerals, is high in chlorophyll, extremely alkaline, detoxifies the body, controls blood glucose, is high in iron, improves blood pressure, decreases constipation, contains valuable enzymes, and is high in protein.
   - *Barley grass:* Another one of nature's super foods. High in minerals, chlorophyll, vitamin A, extremely alkaline, and aids digestion.
   - *Organic green tea:* Loaded with antioxidants and is alkaline.

- *Organic cherry, cranberry or pomegranate juice:* High in antioxidants and naturally detoxifies the body. Mix with mineral water for healthy and refreshing beverages.
- *Sea vegetables:* Sea vegetables such as sushi nori, kelp, and dulse are high in minerals, vitamins, and antioxidants, and detoxify the body.

6. **Frequency:** Three-hour rule
   - Eat small meals frequently (every three hours).
   - Eating frequent small meals improves blood glucose levels, boosts metabolism, and decreases lipase enzyme activity.

7. **Rest/Recovery:**
   - Deep breathing: Take multiple thirty-second deep-breathing breaks throughout the day to relieve stress.
   - Belly breathing.
   - Set up sleep habits: Ideally, get seven to eight hours of sleep per night.
   - Quiet time.
   - Soft music.
   - Regular vacations.
   - Develop rituals for rest, rejuvenation, and recovery.
   - Proper rest and recovery improve health and energy and hormonal and pH balance.

8. **Exercise:**
   - *Dynamic warm-up:* two to three minutes daily
   - *Foundation exercises:* five minutes daily
   - *Cardiovascular exercise:* fifteen to twenty-five minutes, two to seven days a week
   - *Strength training:* five to forty-five minutes, two to seven days a week
   - *Stretching and flexibility:* five to ten minutes daily

9. **Fun:** Find activities you enjoy!

I find change can be difficult but also exciting. A few lifestyle changes that I have recently implemented are deep-breathing exercises three or four times per day, taking frozen wheat grass cubes in the morning and barley grass cubes in the evening, along with organic extra-virgin coconut oil in the evening. I even started drinking green tea on occasion. Now that sounds exciting! Use the *Food Target* to help guide your choices. Experiment with different foods and tastes. Remember, you are the driver of this bus.

Chapter 29
YOU CAN DO IT!

Here's the real challenge: how do you make healthy lifestyle changes a reality? Change is a process and, in most cases, happens in small increments. For some people, the concept of *On Target Living Nutrition* might be initially overwhelming. It may seem too difficult to implement into their lives, because

> ## Slow and steady wins the race.
> —Aesop

there is a great deal of information to absorb at one time. This is why it is important to break it down into steps that you can easily handle.

This section gives you suggestions for where and how you could begin your journey to a healthier lifestyle. Make your decision, develop your plan of action, and DO IT! After you have made a few small changes and are ready for more, go back and read another chapter and begin to make a few more adjustments.

The people whose testimonials you've read in this book did not make their changes overnight. They moved along the continuum, gathering information and making small adjustments until they reached their goals. Make On Target Living your own. Take that first step and never look back!

FINAL TIPS FOR SUCCESS

The law of attraction

The older I get, the more I realize what you focus on is what you will attract into your life. This is the law of attraction! I have become such a believer in this law, especially over the past few years. The "be careful what you wish for because you might get it" is so true. I focus my attention on what I want, not on what I don't want. If I start to focus on what I don't want, I have to stop myself and say, "Is there a better question that I could ask that gets me in the direction I want to go?" It's like the golfer standing on the first tee and not wanting to hit the ball into the water. We all know where the ball is going—in the water! What if the golfer focused on taking slow, deep breaths, making a nice, smooth swing and visualizing the ball going right down the middle of the fairway? Would the outcome be different?

If you had a goal of losing fifty pounds and all you did was focus on how much you dislike being overweight, or you dislike exercise, or you don't like to diet, where will you land? You may be attracting into your life exactly what you don't want. What if you started asking better questions: "How can I be lean and fit and enjoy the process?" "How do I make exercise more enjoyable?" Do you like to dance, ride a bike, or walk? What does it feel like to move your body? Exercise can be so rewarding. Maybe in the past you placed your attention on how you were depriving yourself by eating healthier and giving up certain unhealthy food choices. What if, instead, you placed your attention on what you would get by eating healthier? Your skin starts to look soft and smooth, you have more energy, and you feel stronger with more vitality. Visualize what you want in your life and go after it. What you place your attention on is what you will attract into your life; this is the "law of attraction."

Believe to achieve

We all have areas in our life in which we excel—playing the piano, reading, math, science, skiing, golf, tennis, cooking, listening, speaking, swimming, writing... the list goes on and on. You slowly build confidence by having small successes.

I remember my sixth-grade teacher, Miss Ellis, telling me over and over, "You can be anything you want to be in this world!" As I look back, she probably said this to all of her students. But you know what? It worked. She used to tell me what a great speller I was, and to this day I feel I am a pretty good speller. For some reason I don't remember her telling me I was good in math. Anyway, Miss Ellis, like so many other wonderful teaches in our world, got her students to believe in themselves. You never know how one person can touch another person's life. Thank you, Miss Ellis, for touching my life!

One of my goals when working with personal training clients is to get them to focus on their success, whether it's eating breakfast in the morning, drinking more water at work, moving their bodies more often, lowering their cholesterol, feeling less pain when they get out of bed in the morning, or skiing for the first time in twenty years! No matter how small or large their successes, I want them to make sure that they notice them. My goal is to build their confidence. If they start having a little success their confidence grows and they begin to believe.

Have you ever truly known something would work and it did? You believed it was going to work. No second-guessing or doubt. Is it possible to place disbelief aside? One of my long-time personal training clients, Bob Cornwell, who I call "Pocket Hercules," was discussing the power of belief. At the age of fifty-five Bob is in great shape and has a real passion for health and fitness. Bob is professional pianist and teacher, but those lucky students who get to study and work with Bob know Bob is also a teacher of life! Bob teaches and inspires his students to become better human beings; I believe this is Bob's true gift. When Bob and I get together we like to share strategies between our professions. I have learned so much from Bob over the years and I am extremely grateful for his wisdom and friendship.

Bob told me about a trip he once took with his family to the Field Museum in Chicago. One of the highlights of the museum's Egyptian display was an interactive setup to teach youngsters about the day-to-day life of the ancient Egyptians. Bob's seven-year-old daughter, Sasha, and her friends swarmed over the various installations while he and his wife rested their aching feet.

Pumps, tools, and other objects got the once-over, but a nearby monolithic cube of limestone (indicating the size of a typical block of stone from the Great Pyramid) was all but ignored. As Sasha passed it, she gave the enormous rope with which it was bound a half-hearted tug. Unable to resist, Bob let out a gasp, "I don't believe it!"

"Don't believe what?" Sasha asked."

"It moved!"

Galvanized, Sasha clapped onto the rope and pulled with all her might. As if by magic, her friends and several nearby children, infected by her conviction, took hold and heaved. A chain reaction set in and soon the cube swarmed with little bodies heaving in unison with all their hearts. The chuckles of amused onlookers suddenly changed to gasps as briefly, but unmistakably, the monolith moved.

Later, as he reflected on the incident, what really struck Bob the most was not the surprise of the adults, but the utter certainty of the children. They truly believed. Make small changes, grow your confidence, build on your successes, and believe in yourself and others. We all need more Miss Ellises in this world.

TAKE IT FROM ME...

As a pianist and teacher, my primary goal is to find and use what works. As I explore and discard different approaches to playing a particular passage or communicating a certain concept, I have learned to listen for the "click"; it's the sound a key makes as it turns and opens a lock. I suppose it was this mindset that led me to On Target Living. Inept at sports and increasingly overweight (I had to shop for clothes in the "husky" section, an activity I came to dread), I would periodically starve myself and exercise until I felt sick. Discouraged, I would give up and lose whatever gains I had made. It wasn't until I began training with Chris that I learned to make incremental changes in my food choices and in my approach to exercise, that I felt the key

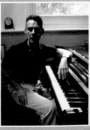

Bob Cornwell

turn in the lock. My energy level and attitude soared and I no longer needed to visit the "husky" section! What had been an ordeal is now an adventure and I've never looked back, fifteen years after hearing that "click."

Expect bumps in the road

We all have times in our lives when we get off track. Don't let one meal, day, week, or even a month of poor eating and exercise habits get you down. Everyone has lapses now and then. Don't give up. Get your focus back. Look at your successes and how you have made improvements along the ladder of health. Even if you have a lapse occasionally, rarely will you go back to where you started. Monitor yourself weekly. Are you getting enough rest? Are you moving your body regularly? Are you making good nutritional decisions? If you have slipped a little, recognize the early warning signs and get back on track toward better health.

ENJOY THE JOURNEY!

I hope you have enjoyed *On Target Living Nutrition*. As with any challenge, the journey is as rewarding as the outcome. Put your back-burner dreams on the front burner. You may be surprised at what you can accomplish. Enjoy the journey—you are worth it!

Health and happiness!—*CJ*

The Two Wolves

One evening an old Cherokee told his grandson about a battle that goes on inside people. He said, "My son, it is between two wolves.

"One is evil. It is anger, envy, sorrow, regret, greed, arrogance, self-pity, guilt, resentment, inferiority, lies, false pride, superiority, ego…

"The other is good. It is joy, peace, love, hope, serenity, humility, kindness, benevolence, empathy, generosity, truth, compassion, and faith."

The grandson thought about it for a minute and then asked his grandfather, "Which wolf wins?"

The old Cherokee simply replied, "The one you feed."

Peace.

Appendix A
ON TARGET LIVING RECIPES

The recipes in this section introduce some healthy alternatives to traditional ingredients. Some of these recipes are original and others are adaptations. Use these recipes as a start, then experiment with your own favorites to convert them into more healthy versions. If you would like more recipes to choose from, pick up a copy of my *On Target Living Cooking* with over 250 great-tasting, healthy recipes!

> ## Forgiveness is the key to action and freedom.
>
> —Hannah Arendt

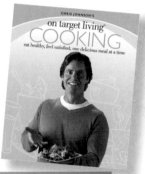

Don't forget, food preparation does not have to be complicated. Baked vegetables drizzled with extra-virgin olive oil or an apple with almond butter are simple and wonderful.

Enjoy these recipe ideas, and then let your imagination fly!

BREAKFAST

CJ's oatmeal on-the-run (cold, uncooked)

Serves 1
526 calories per serving; 47g CHO; 29g FAT; 13g PRO 10g fiber

½	cup rolled oats
1½	tablespoons fresh or frozen fruit
1	tablespoon slivered almonds
2	teaspoons lemon-flavored cod liver oil
1	tablespoon flaxseed oil
½	cup soy milk or organic skim milk
1	dash ground cinnamon

Place all ingredients in a small bowl with lid. Let stand in refrigerator overnight or for ten minutes prior to eating. No cooking required. Fast, easy, healthy, and tastes great!

CJ's granola

13 cups
¼ cup = 102 calories; 16g CHO; 3g FAT; 3g PRO; 3g fiber

6	tablespoons water
2	teaspoons Stevia Plus™ blend
3	tablespoons extra-virgin coconut oil, melted
½	teaspoon sea salt
1	tablespoon vanilla extract
9	cups rolled oats
¾	cup raw, sliced almonds and sunflower seeds
½	cup ground flaxseeds
1	tablespoon cinnamon
½	teaspoon ground nutmeg
2¼	cups chopped dried apples
¾	cup chopped prunes

Preheat oven to 275°. In small bowl, mix water, Stevia Plus™, coconut oil, salt, and vanilla; set aside. In large bowl, mix oats, almonds, ground flaxseeds, cinnamon, and nutmeg. Pour water mixture over oats mixture. Stir to blend thoroughly. Spread on cookie sheet. Bake 45–60 minutes, stirring two times. Remove from oven and cool thoroughly. Add dried fruits. Refrigerate to keep flaxseeds fresh. Use as a cold cereal with milk, as a cooked cereal (½ cup granola cooked for seven minutes with ¾ to 1 cup water), or as a snack.

scrambled eggs

Serves 2
230 calories per serving; 10g CHO; 14g FAT; 16g PRO; 3g fiber

2   egg whites (free-range)
2   whole eggs (free-range)
1   large garlic clove, minced
1   tablespoon chopped fresh oregano
½   red bell pepper, diced
½   green bell pepper, diced
½   small white onion, diced
½   tablespoon extra-virgin olive oil
    sea salt and freshly ground black pepper, to taste
1   tablespoon grated low-fat cheddar or swiss cheese

Whisk eggs and herbs in medium bowl. Stir in peppers and onion. Lightly coat a medium skillet with olive oil and heat over medium heat. Pour egg mixture into skillet. Add garlic, oregano, salt, and pepper; scramble until cooked. Sprinkle with cheddar or swiss cheese.

Variation: Replace vegetable mixture with:
1   cup broccoli florets
½   cup sliced yellow or zucchini squash
⅓   cup corn
2   ounces cooked, uncured, nitrate-free turkey ham, chopped

oatmeal pancakes

10 pancakes, Serves 3–4
1 pancake = 98 calories; 15g CHO; 2g FAT; 5g PRO; 2g fiber (excluding fruit topping)

2	tablespoons soy milk
5	egg whites (free-range)
2	whole eggs (free-range)
1½	cups rolled oats
½	cup low-fat cottage cheese
½	cup natural unsweetened applesauce
½	teaspoon vanilla extract
½	teaspoon cinnamon
½	tablespoon extra-virgin olive oil

Mix all ingredients except oil in a blender until smooth (add more milk for creamier batter). Pour into large bowl; let stand for 5 minutes. Pour ⅓ cup batter per pancake onto hot, oiled griddle. Cook until bubbles form, then flip. Serve topped with a spoonful of fruit or natural applesauce.

SNACKS

energized bars

12 bars
1 bar = 200 calories; 33g CHO; 4g FAT; 8g PRO; 3g fiber

1	20-ounce can crushed pineapple in own juice
½	cup crushed almonds
2	cups rolled oats
3	scoops hemp, rice, soy, or whey protein powder
1	cup chopped dried fruit
1½	teaspoons cinnamon

Preheat oven to 200°. Combine all ingredients. Spread in 13×9-inch pan brushed with expeller-pressed canola oil or almond oil. Bake for 90 minutes. Cool and slice. Store in refrigerator. Great snack anytime.

CJ's smoothie

Serves 3 (16 ounces each)
194 calories per serving; 24g CHO; 6g FAT; 11g PRO; 12g fiber

- 3   cups filtered water
- 2   scoops soy, rice, hemp, or whey protein powder
- 1   16-ounce bag frozen unsweetened fruit
- 1   banana
- 1½   tablespoons flaxseed oil or flax meal

Combine ingredients in blender. Cover and blend at high speed about
1 minute. Keep refrigerated until served.

flax bran muffins

Serves 12
1 muffin = 233 calories; 34g CHO; 8g FAT; 8g PRO; 6g fiber

- 1½   cups white whole wheat flour (unbleached, unbromated)
- ¾   cup ground flaxseeds
- ¾   cup oat bran
- ¼   cup brown sugar + 3 tablespoons Stevia Plus™
- 2   teaspoons baking soda
- 1   teaspoon aluminum-free baking powder
- ½   teaspoon sea salt
- 2   teaspoons cinnamon
- 1½   cups shredded carrots
- 2   apples, unpeeled, shredded
- ½   cup raisins
- ¾   cup chopped walnuts
- 3   egg whites (free-range)
- ¾   cup soy milk
- 1   teaspoon vanilla extract

Preheat oven to 350°. Combine flour, flaxseeds, oat bran, sugar, baking
soda, baking powder, salt and cinnamon in a large bowl and mix well. Add
carrots, apples, raisins and nuts. In a separate bowl, blend egg whites, milk
and vanilla. Add liquid ingredients to dry ingredients; mix until just
combined. Do not over stir. Coat muffin tin with coconut oil. Divide mixture
into 12 muffin cups. Bake for 27–30 minutes. Allow to cool slightly; remove
from muffin tin to finish cooling.

SALADS

cherry chicken salad

Serves 4
264 calories per serving; 12g CHO; 12g FAT; 27g PRO; 3g fiber

1   pound boneless, skinless, chicken breast (grilled, poached, steamed, or pan-seared), cut into 1-inch cubes
½   cup dried cherries
¼   cup canola mayonnaise blended with ½ teaspoon prepared mustard
¼   cup broken walnuts
¾   cup diagonally sliced celery
⅛   cup chopped onion

Mix all ingredients. Serve on a bed of greens or fill a whole-grain tortilla for a wrap sandwich.

black bean mango salad

6 cups
1 cup = 214 calories; 32g CHO; 6g FAT; 8g PRO; 10g fiber

2   15-ounce cans black beans, rinsed and drained
1½   cups fresh or frozen corn, cooked
½   green bell pepper, chopped
½   red bell pepper, chopped
4   green onions, sliced thin
1   avocado, cubed
1   mango, cubed
2   tablespoons extra-virgin olive oil
2   tablespoons balsamic vinegar

Mix all ingredients together. Refrigerate for 1 hour. One of my favorites.

CJ's big salad

Serves 1
367 calories per serving; 24g CHO; 19g FAT; 25g PRO; 8g fiber

| 1 | tablespoons balsamic vinegar
| 1 | tablespoon extra-virgin olive oil
| ½ | cup broccoli slaw
| 5 | grape tomatoes
| 2 | cups spinach or Romaine lettuce, torn
| ⅛ | cup sliced red pepper
| 1 | tablespoon raisins or dried cherries
| ½ | tablespoon slivered almonds
| 1 | 6-ounce can tuna or wild salmon in water

Mix vinegar and oil together; set aside. Mix all other ingredients in a large bowl. Drizzle vinegar and oil mixture over top of salad; toss. This is my lunch two or three times per week; fast, easy, healthy, and I love the taste.

salmon salad

Serves 4
346 calories per serving; 18g CHO; 18g FAT; 28g PRO; 3g fiber

| 8 | tablespoons extra-virgin olive oil, divided
| 4 | tablespoons balsamic vinegar
| | sea salt and freshly ground black pepper to taste
| ¼ | cup vegetable, chicken, or fish broth
| 4 | 4-ounce salmon fillets
| 6 | cups spinach or Romaine lettuce
| 2 | tablespoons capers, drained
| ½ | small red onion, thinly sliced
| 4 | tablespoons cooked corn kernels

In a small bowl, whisk together 6 tablespoons oil and 3 tablespoons vinegar. Season with salt and pepper and set aside to use as dressing. Pour remaining oil and vinegar into a large sauté pan; add broth. Heat to a boil, reduce temperature, and add salmon. Cover pan, poach for 10–15 minutes, and then transfer to a plate to cool. Prepare each serving plate with 1½ cups of greens. Add salmon fillet and garnish with capers, red onion, and corn. Drizzle balsamic vinaigrette over each serving.

DRESSINGS/DIPS

so simple salad dressing

Serves 16
2 tablespoons = 116 calories; 2g CHO; 12g FAT; 0g PRO; 0g fiber

- 1   cup extra-virgin olive oil
- 1   cup balsamic vinegar (or vinegar of choice)

Mix with a wire whisk. Store at room temperature. Always ready to serve.

caesar salad dressing

12 tablespoons
3 tablespoons dressing = 65 calories; 1g CHO; 5g FAT; 2g PRO; 0g fiber

- ⅓   cup low-fat sour cream
- ¼   cup canola mayonnaise
- 1   tablespoon grated Parmesan cheese
- 2   tablespoons chopped Italian flat leaf parsley
- 1   tablespoon skim milk
- ½   teaspoon freshly ground black pepper
- ½   teaspoon Worcestershire sauce
- 1   tablespoon lemon juice
- 2   garlic cloves, minced
- ¼   teaspoon anchovy paste

Mix ingredients in a small bowl and whisk to blend well. Set aside until ready to dress salad.

SOUPS/CHILIS

fast chicken noodle soup

10 cups
1 cup = 121 calories; 9g CHO; 5g FAT; 12g PRO; 2g fiber

1	tablespoon extra-virgin olive oil
1	cup diced celery
1	cup chopped onion
1½	cups chopped carrots
2	garlic cloves, minced
8	cups chicken broth
½	teaspoon sea salt
	freshly ground black pepper
½	teaspoon dried thyme, crushed
¼	teaspoon dried oregano, crushed
½	teaspoon poultry seasoning
1	pound boneless, skinless chicken breast
1	cup (2 ounces) fine whole-wheat noodles
1	cup frozen green peas

In large skillet, heat olive oil over medium-high heat; sauté celery, onion, carrots, and garlic for 5 minutes. Add broth, salt, pepper, thyme, oregano, poultry seasoning, and chicken. Bring to boil; reduce heat, cover, and simmer for 5 minutes. Uncover and return broth to a boil. Add noodles and peas and bring to a boil again. Reduce heat, cover, and simmer for 12 minutes. Remove chicken from broth and cut into cubes; return chicken to broth; heat through. Ready to serve. (Freezes well.)

ostrich soup

Serves 6
336 calories per serving; 25g CHO; 12g FAT; 32g PRO; 5g fiber

2	teaspoons extra-virgin olive oil
1½	pounds ground ostrich
1	onion, chopped
1	green bell pepper, chopped
½	red bell pepper, chopped
4	garlic cloves, minced
32	ounces tomato purée
32	ounces filtered water
2	cups sliced green beans
2	cups chopped kale or spinach
1	cup chopped celery
	sea salt and freshly ground black pepper, to taste

Heat oil in a soup pot over medium heat. Add meat and brown, stirring to separate meat particles and incorporate brown bits. Add onion, bell peppers, and garlic; cook until tender (about 5 minutes). Add remaining ingredients and simmer for 20 minutes. This is an excellent tasting, nutritious soup. Give it a try.

sweet potato minestrone

10 5 cups
I cup = 184 calories; 23g CHO; 5g FAT; IIg PRO; 5g fiber

2	teaspoons extra-virgin olive oil
½	pound lean ground turkey
I	cup sliced onion
I	cup diced carrots
¾	cup thinly sliced celery
3	cups chicken broth
2	cups peeled, diced sweet potato
2	14.5-ounce cans no-salt-added whole tomatoes, chopped, undrained
I	15-ounce can great northern beans, rinsed and drained
I	teaspoon dried oregano
½	teaspoon freshly ground black pepper
¼	teaspoon sea salt
8	cups coarsely chopped spinach

Heat olive oil in a large saucepan over medium-high heat. Add meat, onion, carrots, and celery, and sauté for 7 minutes, stirring to separate meat particles and incorporate brown bits, or until meat is browned. Add broth and all remaining ingredients, except spinach. Bring to a boil; cover, reduce heat, and simmer for 15 minutes or until vegetables are tender. Stir in spinach; cook an additional 2 minutes.

white chicken chili

10 cups
1 cup = 128 calories; 11g CHO; 4g FAT; 12g PRO; 3g fiber

- 1 tablespoon extra-virgin olive oil
- 1 large onion, chopped
- 1 red or green pepper, chopped
- 2 garlic cloves, minced
- 1 15-ounce can white beans, rinsed and drained
- 3 cups chicken broth, divided
- 2 cups cooked chicken breast, cubed
- 1 14.5-ounce can Italian stewed tomatoes
- 2 teaspoons chili powder
- 1 teaspoon cumin
- 1 teaspoon dried oregano
  sea salt and freshly ground black pepper, to taste
- 1 ounce (¼ cup) reduced-fat cheese, shredded (optional)

In large skillet, heat olive oil over medium-high heat and sauté onion, pepper, and garlic for 3–5 minutes. Meanwhile, put 1 cup of beans and 1½ cups chicken broth in blender, and blend until smooth. Add all the beans, chicken, remaining broth, and seasonings to skillet. Simmer for 15 minutes. Serve in bowls, each sprinkled with 1 tablespoon reduced-fat shredded cheese. (Best if made ahead and allowed to steep; freezes well.)

ENTRÉES

buffalo/turkey meatloaf

Serves 8
187 calories per serving; 10g CHO; 6g FAT; 16g PRO; 4g fiber

1	medium onion, finely chopped
1	medium carrot, finely chopped
4	medium mushrooms, finely chopped
1	garlic clove, minced
½	cup cooked beans or lentils, mashed
8	ounces ground turkey breast
8	ounces ground buffalo
¾	cup salsa, divided
1	egg (free-range)
¼	cup skim milk
¾	teaspoon Italian herb mix
¼	teaspoon sea salt
	freshly ground black pepper
½	tablespoon regular mustard
½	tablespoon Worcestershire sauce
2	tablespoons extra-virgin olive oil
¾	cup rolled oats

Preheat oven to 350°. Put meats in a medium bowl. Add chopped vegetables, mashed beans, ½ cup of salsa, and remaining ingredients. Mix thoroughly. Lightly coat a 9×4-inch bread pan with olive oil and shape meatloaf in pan. Bake for 35 minutes. Spread remaining ¼ cup salsa on top of meatloaf and continue baking 35 minutes more or until internal temperature is 160°. Do not overbake.

chicken and vegetable pizza

8 slices
I slice = 230 calories; 23g CHO; 8g FAT; 21g PRO; 4g fiber

- | pound boneless, skinless chicken breast, cut in ½-inch cubes
- | tablespoon extra-virgin olive oil
- | small onion, sliced
- ½   green bell pepper, sliced
- ½   red bell pepper, sliced
- ⅓   cup mango, pineapple, peach chutney, or salsa
- | 8-ounce can pineapple tidbits, drained
- | cup (4 ounces) shredded reduced-fat mozzarella cheese
- | 12-inch, ready-made, thin whole-grain pizza crust

Preheat oven to 450°. Heat oil in large skillet; sauté chicken, onion, and peppers until chicken is no longer pink. Spread chutney evenly on ready-made pizza crust. Spread chicken mixture and pineapple tidbits over chutney and sprinkle cheese on top. Bake for 10–12 minutes and cut into 8 slices.

salmon or tuna patties

Serves 4 or 5
274 calories per serving; 16g CHO; 12g FAT; 26g PRO; 2g fiber

- | 16-ounce can salmon or tuna
- | teaspoon lemon juice
- ½   cup chopped onion
- ½   cup chopped celery
- 4   egg whites (free-range)
- ⅔   cup whole-grain bread crumbs
- 2   tablespoons soy milk
- 2   tablespoons extra-virgin olive oil

Drain salmon or tuna. Discard bones and skin and flake meat. Combine fish with lemon juice, onion, celery, egg whites, ⅓ cup bread crumbs, and milk; mix well. Shape into 4 or 5 patties and coat with remaining bread crumbs. In large skillet, heat oil over medium heat. Cook patties about 3 minutes or until browned. Carefully turn with metal spatula and brown other side about 3 minutes more.

salmon teriyaki

Serves 6
216 calories per serving; 6g CHO; 10g FAT; 27g PRO; 2g fiber (excluding rice or potatoes)

- 2 pounds wild-caught salmon fillets
- 8 fresh green onions (including green tops), chopped
- 12 slices fresh gingerroot
- ½ cup light teriyaki sauce or Bragg's Liquid Aminos™
- 2 cups steamed brown rice

Preheat oven to 425°. Place salmon in shallow baking dish, skin side down. Sprinkle with onions, scatter gingerroot slices, and pour teriyaki or Bragg's over the salmon. Cover tightly with aluminum foil. Bake 20 minutes or until fish flakes easily with a fork. Serve with ½ cup steamed brown rice or two small redskin potatoes.

baked eggplant

Serves 6
210 calories per serving; 27g CHO; 2g FAT; 21g PRO; 6g fiber (not including rice)

- 1 tablespoon extra-virgin olive oil
- 1 pound lean ground turkey
- 2 medium onions, chopped
- ½ teaspoon sea salt
- ½ teaspoon freshly ground black pepper
- ½ teaspoon ground allspice
- ½ teaspoon cinnamon
- 3 large eggplants, peeled and cut into ½-inch slices
- 1 15-ounce can tomato purée
- 3 cups steamed brown rice

In large skillet, heat olive oil over medium heat and brown turkey, stirring to separate meat particles. A onion and seasonings, sauté an additional 5 minutes, and set aside. Broil or sauté eggplant in large skillet until tender. Preheat oven to 375°. In a 9×13-inch pan, layer eggplant then turkey mixture. Pour tomato purée over all. Bake for 20–25 minutes or until bubbly. Serve over ½ cup steamed brown rice.

VEGETABLES AND SIDES

roasted sweet potato wedges

Serves 4
150 calories per serving; 24g CHO; 5g FAT; 2g PRO; 3g fiber

1	pound pared sweet potatoes (2 large), each cut into 8 lengthwise wedges
1½	tablespoons extra-virgin olive oil
½	teaspoon sea salt

Lightly coat a cookie sheet with olive oil. Place potato wedges on cookie sheet and sprinkle with olive oil and sea salt. Lay wedges on one cut side. Bake at 425° for 15 minutes. Turn each wedge to its other cut side for even caramelizing, and bake another 15 minutes. Fresh vegetables may be added to roast for the last 10–15 minutes.

greek tomato salad

6 cups
1 cup = 103 calories; 12g CHO; 6g FAT; 3g PRO; 3g fiber

¼	cup red wine vinegar
2	tablespoons extra-virgin olive oil
2	garlic cloves, minced
½	teaspoon dried oregano
¼	teaspoon dried basil
	sea salt and freshly ground black pepper, to taste
1	cup thinly sliced red onion, rings quartered
1	green pepper, cut in 1-inch chunks
6	medium unpeeled tomatoes, each cut into 8 wedges, then halved
6	medium pitted whole ripe olives, halved
3	tablespoons crumbled feta cheese

In a medium bowl, whisk together vinegar, olive oil, garlic, oregano, basil, salt, and pepper. Add prepared vegetables, olives, and cheese. Cover and let sit on the counter for at least 1 hour to season; stir occasionally to blend flavors. Great on bed of Romaine lettuce. Refrigerate leftovers.

Variation: Add 12 spears of asparagus that have been cut into 1-inch pieces, steamed, placed in ice water to prevent further cooking, and drained.

DESSERTS

cookies that "rock"

48 cookies
89 calories per serving; 11g CHO; 4g FAT; 3g PRO 1g fiber (with sugar)
72 calories per serving; 7g CHO; 4g FAT; 3g PRO; 1g fiber (with Stevia Plus™)

1	cup whole-wheat flour (unbleached, unbromated)
1	cup rolled oats
¾	cup ground flaxseeds
1	teaspoon cinnamon
1	teaspoon baking soda
1	teaspoon sea salt
1	cup whey protein powder
1	cup packed brown sugar (OR 4 tablespoons Stevia Plus™ blend)
6	egg whites (free-range)
½	cup natural unsweetened applesauce
1	teaspoon almond oil
1	tablespoon vanilla extract
1	cup chocolate chips
¾	cup chopped walnuts

Preheat oven to 350°. Combine dry ingredients, except chocolate chips and nuts, and mix well. Add egg whites, applesauce, oil, and vanilla. Beat with electric mixer until combined. Stir in chocolate chips and nuts. For each cookie, drop 1 rounded teaspoon of dough onto oiled cookie sheet, 2 inches apart, flattening slightly. Bake on middle rack of oven for 6–7 minutes (for soft cookie) to 10 minutes (for crunchy cookie). Transfer cookies to a wire rack to cool. Can be frozen.

carrot cake

Serves 8
283 calories per serving; 33g CHO; 13g FAT; 8g PRO; 5g fiber (with sugar)
253 calories per serving; 26g CHO; 13g FAT; 8g PRO; 5g fiber (with sugar and Stevia Plus™)

2	tablespoons extra-virgin coconut oil, softened
2	eggs (free-range)
¾	cup granulated sugar (OR ⅓ cup sugar + 1½ tablespoons Stevia Plus™ blend)
¼	cup skim milk
½	teaspoon vanilla extract
1	tablespoon cinnamon
½	teaspoon ground nutmeg
1⅓	cups white whole-wheat flour (unbleached, unbromated)
½	cup ground flaxseeds, flax meal, or chopped walnuts
1	teaspoon baking soda
1	teaspoon aluminum-free baking powder
½	teaspoon sea salt
1½	cups grated carrots
½	cup raisins
1	teaspoon orange peel, grated

Preheat oven to 350°. In a large bowl, beat oil, eggs, sugar (and Stevia Plus™, if used), milk, and vanilla with a mixer (or by hand) until creamy. Mix cinnamon, nutmeg, flour, flax (or walnuts, if used), baking soda, baking powder, and salt in a separate bowl; then add to the egg mixture. Beat for an additional minute. Add carrots, raisins, and orange peel; stir until combined. Spoon batter into a lightly oiled 8×8-inch baking pan and bake 30–40 minutes or until done. Cake is done when you touch it lightly in the center, and it springs back.

apple crisp

Serves 8
200 calories per serving; 28g CHO; 8g FAT; 4g PRO; 9g fiber

5   pounds apples, peeled and sliced
2   teaspoons cinnamon
2   cups rolled oats
1   cup whole-wheat flour (unbleached, unbromated)
¼   cup packed brown sugar
¼   teaspoon sea salt
1   teaspoon aluminum-free baking powder
2   eggs (free-range)
½   cup butter, melted

Preheat oven to 325°. Toss apples with cinnamon and arrange in bottom of a 9×13-inch pan. In a medium bowl, mix dry ingredients together. In a small bowl, lightly beat eggs. Add eggs to dry ingredients and gently work in eggs until mixture is crumbly. Sprinkle mixture on top of apples. Pour melted butter evenly over the top. Bake 1 hour.

MISCELLANEOUS

taco seasoning

33 calories per serving; 8g CHO; < .1g FAT; < .1 g PRO; < .1 g fiber
Makes 2 tablespoons, equivalent to using 1 packet of purchased taco seasoning

2   teaspoons instant minced onion
1   teaspoon sea salt
1   teaspoon chili powder
½   teaspoon arrowroot
¼   teaspoon dried red pepper, crushed
½   teaspoon garlic powder
¼   teaspoon dried oregano
½   teaspoon ground cumin

Put in blender or Mini-Mate Cuisinart and pulse 10 times. Store in an airtight container. Use for tacos, southwestern soup, taco salad, refried beans, chicken fajitas, or nachos.

Appendix B
ON TARGET LIVING EXERCISES

This section introduces you to a variety of exercises that can be completed with a minimal investment of time, equipment, or expense. Use the written information on exercise in Chapter 26 along with the photos in this section. I have given you a few sample exercise routines in the back of this section as a start. Try to maintain balance in your exercise program and pay attention to proper form for all exercises. Start slowly and enjoy all the benefits that regular exercise brings.

> Shoot for the moon. Even if you miss it, you will land among the stars.
>
> —Les Brown

POSTURE

Here are a few tips to improve your posture. With every exercise you perform, your first thought should be, "Am I in ideal posture?"

- Place **feet** together or hip width apart, toes pointed straight ahead. Feet should be even with each other with your weight distributed evenly. I like to start most people with their feet together to help feel the muscles of the inner legs and core.
- **Knees** should be straight but not locked (soft knees).
- **Hips** should be level with a neutral pelvis. To find neutral pelvis, rotate hips forward (tuck your tail in), rotate back (stick your glutes out) and end in the middle of these two movements. Abdominal and glute muscles should be engaged for stabilization.
- Lift your **rib cage** (chest) up, pull navel up and in, pull your shoulders back and down.
- Keep your **arms** at your sides with palms facing the body, thumbs pointing straight ahead.
- **Head** and **neck** centered over your shoulders. Keep your eyes straight ahead with chin parallel to the ground.

Practice this posture daily and see what a difference ideal posture can make.

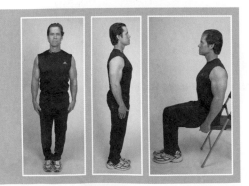

WARM-UP

As with any exercise program you need to make a slow transition from being sedentary to being active. The major goal of the warm-up phase is to increase the temperature of the body allowing greater blood circulation, increasing the temperature of the muscles and connective tissues, and increasing elasticity in the muscles (easier to move and stretch). Your warm-up should last 5–10 minutes. Fast walking or riding a stationary bike are excellent warm-up exercises. If you do not have time to walk or ride a bike, then go directly to dynamic stretching.

Dynamic Stretching

Dynamic stretching is done by actively moving the body in a controlled fashion through the desired range of motion. The major advantage dynamic stretching has over static stretching before you exercise is that it engages the nervous system to activate your muscles, getting them ready to move. Start with the arms and gradually move down the body. Do each exercise slowly and controlled, with 4–10 repetitions per exercise. **Dynamic stretching should take between two and three minutes**.

Arm Swing
Alternate raising arms, palms facing each other.

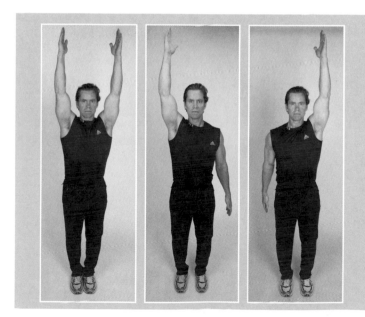

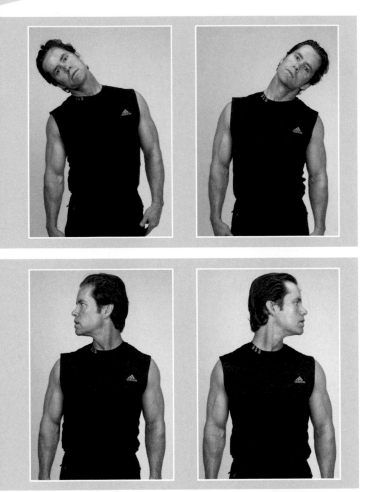

Neck Stretch (Side to Side)

Target Muscles:
Neck and trapezius.
Start with ideal standing posture, keeping shoulders pulled back and down. Tip head to side taking ear directly to shoulder.
Hold stretch 2–3 seconds on each side.

Neck Stretch (Rotation)

Target Muscles:
Neck and trapezius.
Start with ideal standing posture, keeping shoulders pulled back and down. Rotate head side to side, looking in opposite directions.
Hold stretch 2–3 seconds on each side.

Round the Spine

As you round your spine pull navel into your spine.

Side Bend

As you reach over let opposite heel come up. Keep navel pulled up and in.

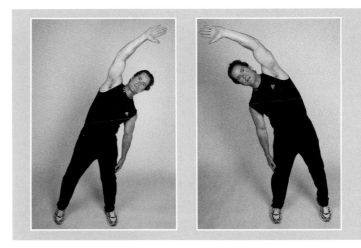

Trunk Twist

As you twist lift heel. Twist slowly side to side. Keep navel pulled up and in.

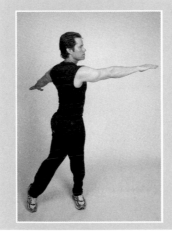
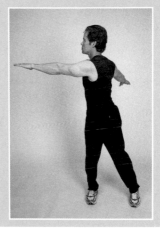

Front Leg Swing

Hold on to the wall or a chair when first performing this exercise. Maintain ideal posture. To improve balance try this exercise without holding on.

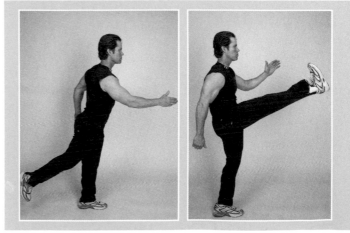

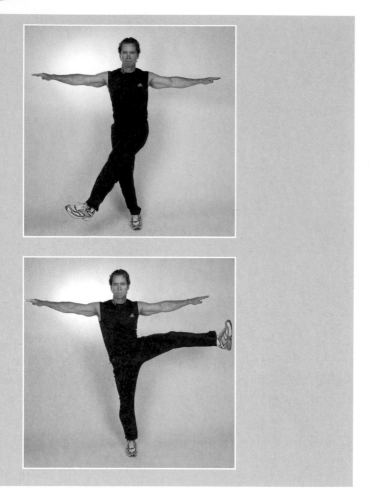

Side Leg Swing

Hold on to the wall or a chair when first performing this exercise. Try to maintain ideal posture. Slight bend in the knee of the support leg and point the toe up in both directions. To improve balance and coordination try this exercise without holding on.

FOUNDATION EXERCISES

Foundation exercises can improve your posture, strength, balance, flexibility, and fitness all at the same time. I wanted to have a series of exercises that could improve my personal training clients' and my own personal fitness in a short amount of time. The beauty of these foundational exercises is that they don't take much time, can be done almost anywhere with no equipment requirements, and, most of all, they work.

I have all of my personal training clients using the foundation exercises in some manner every day. You may choose to modify each movement or add or delete any of the exercises to fit your current needs. You may choose to do foundation exercises before you play golf, tennis, basketball, bike, walk, jog or run, lift weights or just as your main source of exercise for that day. Hold each exercise for five to twenty seconds, and focus on the proper technique for each movement. **Foundation exercises should take 5–7 minutes to complete.**

Standing or Seated Posture

Stand or sit with feet together or hip width apart, weight distributed evenly and hips level. Do not lock knees. Lift your rib cage (chest) up, pull navel up and in, pull your shoulders back and down. Keep your arms at your sides with palms facing the body, thumbs pointing straight ahead. Make sure head and neck are centered over your shoulders. Keep your eyes straight ahead with chin parallel to the ground.

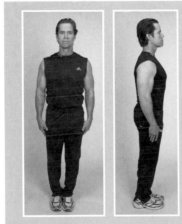

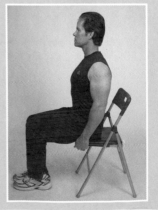

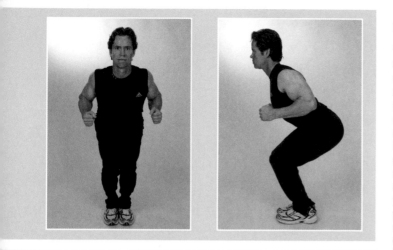

Squat

Target Muscles:
Glutes, quadriceps, and hamstrings.
Start in ideal posture, hands fisted, pull elbows back, navel up and in, and weight spread evenly on your feet. Push hips back and bend forward slowly as you squat. Pause the bend at 90 degrees. Keep knees aligned with second toe. As you slowly stand up, squeeze your glutes. To modify the movement (make it easier) decrease range of motion or hold on to counter or table.

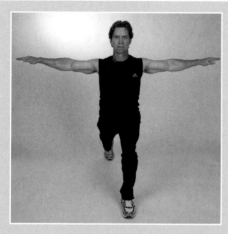

Straight Leg Lunge

Target Muscles:
Quadriceps, glutes, and hamstrings.
Start with feet shoulder width apart. Extend arms out from shoulders while bending the knee to a 90-degree angle and slowly reaching back with the opposite leg to a wide stance lunge. Back leg is straight, glute is contracted (tight). Front leg knee is tracking over the second toe. Pull navel up and in. To create more stability, place hands on a wall. Hold this movement for 10–30 seconds.

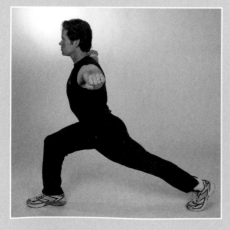

Warrior 3

Target Muscles:

Quadriceps, glutes, feet, shoulders, back, hamstrings, and core.

Begin in ideal posture position with arms raised overhead. Slowly bend at waist while lifting one leg backward to form a "T." Arms may stay extended or at your side. Contract glutes and pull navel up and in. Hold movement. Repeat on opposite side. Warrior 3 is great for balance. Start slowly and watch your balance improve.

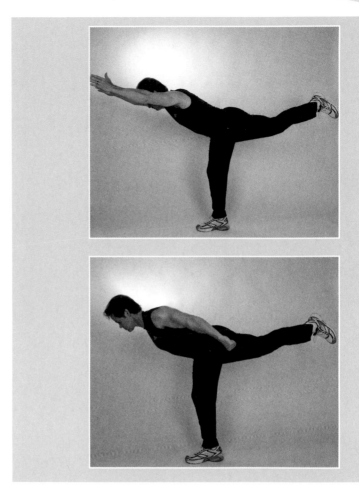

Half Moon

Target Muscles:

Quadriceps, glutes, feet, shoulders, hamstrings, inner thigh, and core.

Start in Warrior 3 and slowly reach down (hand does not touch floor) and reach up with opposite hand and look down. Half moon is great for improving your balance.

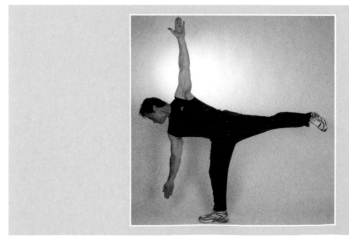

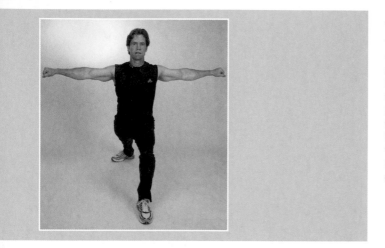

Warrior 1

Target Muscles:
Glutes, quads, hamstrings, core, inner thighs, back, and feet.
Line up the heel of your front foot with the arch of your back foot. Extend arms out from the shoulders while bending the front knee to a 90-degree angle. Your back leg is straight, glutes and navel engaged, with chest up.

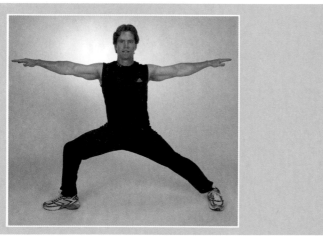

Warrior 2

Target Muscles:
Glutes, quadriceps, hamstrings, core, inner thighs, back, and feet.
Same position as Warrior 1 except you rotate your body. Keep your front knee lined up with the second toe, keep back leg straight, keep your core engaged.

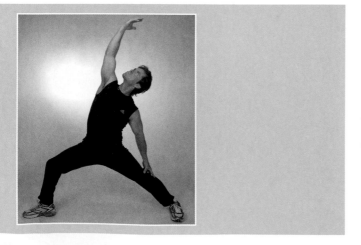

Reverse Warrior

Target Muscles:
Glutes, quadriceps, hamstrings, core, inner thighs, back, and feet.
Same position as Warrior 2. Place hand on the knee of the back leg, reach up and back with opposite hand, palm of hand facing in, look up to your hand.

Extended Angle

Target Muscles:

Adductors, quadriceps, glutes, shoulders, back, core, and feet.
Square up front foot, align knee over the second toe, back foot turned in 3–4 inches. Lunge forward, keeping the weight centered over the front foot and on the outside of the back foot. Reaching forward, place hand on your knee or at the base of the foot on the floor. Reach up with opposite arm and open up shoulders and chest. Squeeze glutes and pull navel up and in. A great rotational stretch, especially for those who play golf, tennis, racquetball, squash, or handball.

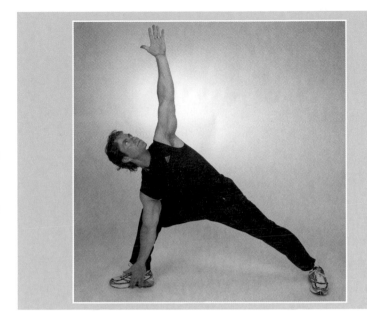

Spread Eagle

Target Muscles:

Adductors, quadriceps, glutes, core, and feet.
Spread legs apart, toes pointed straight forward, knees slightly bent, arms out to side, chest up, flat back, and sink glutes toward the floor.

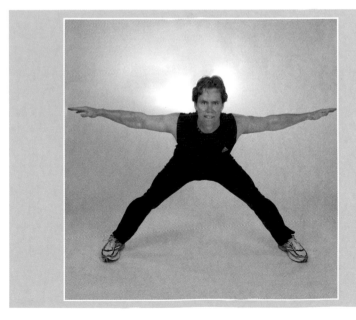

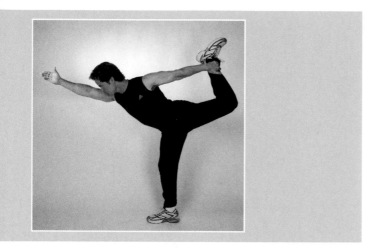

Dancer

Target Muscles:

Quadriceps, glutes, feet, shoulders, back, hamstrings, and core.

Grab ankle or top of foot with one arm and extend the other arm overhead. Slowly bend at waist. Keep knee of stabilizing leg slightly bent. Try to pull the foot away from your glute. Contract glutes, pull navel up and in. Hold movement. Repeat on opposite side.

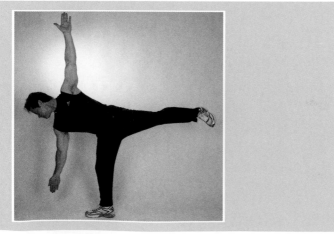

Wall Posture— Thoracic Extensions

Target Muscles:

Middle and upper back, shoulders, core, and legs.

Stand with feet and knees together, bend knees. Head back of shoulders and glutes touch the wall, look straight ahead. Hands face in, arms straight, reach up. Contract your ankles, calves, inner thighs, glutes, and navel up and in. You can modify using one arm only.

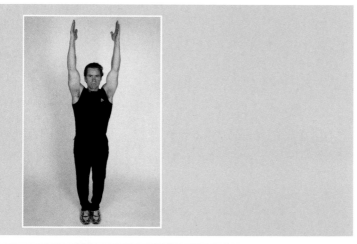

Half Moon

Target Muscles:

Quadriceps, glutes, feet, shoulders, back, inner thigh, and hamstrings.

Place front foot 4–5 inches away from the wall. Go up on one leg, lean against the wall, reach down and reach up. Palms face out. Look up to hand. Great for balance and flexibility in your back, shoulders, neck, and inner thigh.

Standing Downward Dog

Target Muscles:
Full body.
Hold onto a fixed object, feet shoulder width apart. Push hips back and push shoulders toward floor. Keep back, head, and arms in neutral alignment. Modify stretch by slightly bending knees. A great stretch that is easy to perform and can be done virtually anywhere.

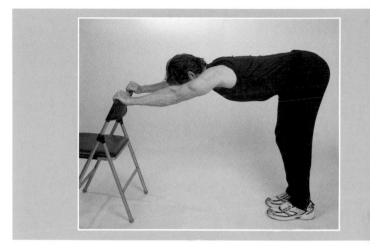

Standing Upward Dog

Target Muscles:
Full body.
Feet shoulder width apart, place hands on fixed object, face forward, chest up, glutes tight, pull navel up and in. Slowly pull hips forward, head back, shoulders down and in.

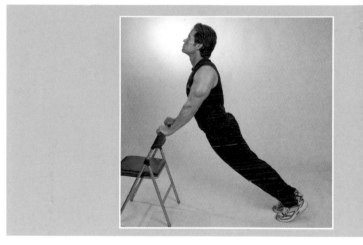

STRENGTH TRAINING

Strength training is exercise that uses resistance to place demands on the nervous system, hormones, bones, and muscles. The benefits of strength training include increased strength, increased bone density, improved mobility and functionality, improved posture, better balance, fewer injuries, improved athletic performance, reduced stress, increased self-esteem, increased metabolism, and weight control.

Strength training is generally done with a short burst (ten to thirty seconds) of the strength training phase, followed by a recovery phase. The rest or recovery phase can last ten seconds to four minutes, depending on your goals.

Lower Body

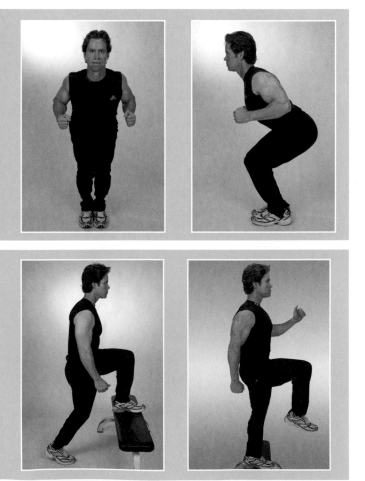

Squat

Target Muscles:
Glutes, quadriceps, hamstrings, core, and back.

Start in ideal posture, hands fisted, pull elbows back, navel up and in, and weight spread evenly on your feet. Push hips back and bend forward slowly as you squat. Pause the bend at 90 degrees. Keep knees aligned with second toe. As you slowly stand up, squeeze your glutes. To modify the movement (make it easier) decrease range of motion or hold on to counter or table.

Step-up

Target Muscles:
Quadriceps, glutes, hamstrings, core, and back.

Place feet on a solid bench or step (something that does not move). Keep weight evenly distributed in the front foot, step up slowly bringing your knee up with the opposite arm. Step down slowly. Excellent for strength, fitness, and balance.

Straight Leg Lunge

Target Muscles:
*Quadriceps, glutes,
and hamstrings.*
Start with feet shoulder width
apart. Extend arms out from
shoulders while bending the
knee to a 90-degree angle
and slowly reaching back with
the opposite leg to a wide
stance lunge. Back leg is
straight, glute is contracted
(tight). Front leg knee is
tracking over the second toe.
Pull navel up and in. Don't
forget to breathe. Hold this
movement for 10–30 seconds.

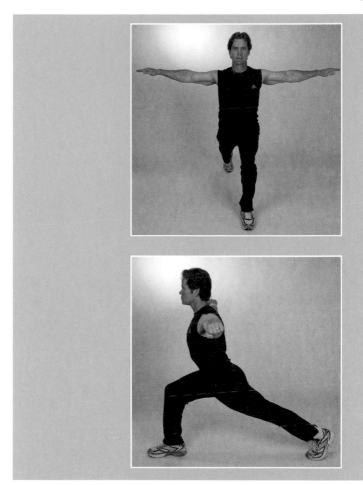

Warrior I

Target Muscles:
*Glutes, quads, hamstrings, core,
inner thighs, back, and feet.*
Line up the heel of your front
foot with the arch of your
back foot. Extend arms out
from the shoulders while
bending the front knee to a
90-degree angle. Your back
leg is straight, glutes and navel
engaged, with chest up.

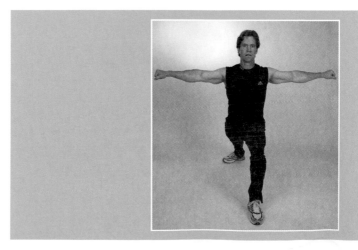

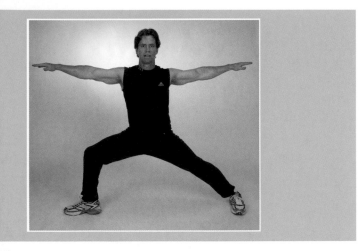

Warrior 2

Target Muscles:
Glutes, quadriceps, hamstrings, core, inner thighs, back, and feet.
Same position as Warrior 1 except you rotate your body. Keep your front knee lined up with the second toe, keep back leg straight, keep your core engaged.

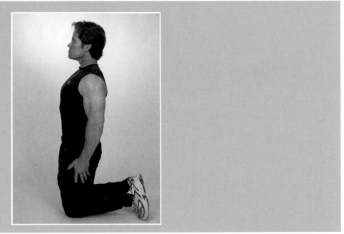

Kneeling Hamstring

Target Muscles:
Hamstrings, glutes, core, back, and posture.
Place knees on a pillow or soft mat. Pull ankles, calves, hamstrings, and glutes together. Navel up and in, chest up, shoulders down and in. Contract muscles for 10–15 seconds. Repeat 3–5 times.

Supine Hip Extension

Target Muscles:
Hamstrings, glutes, core, back, and posture.
If you can't place pressure on your knees, this exercise can substitute for the kneeling hamstring exercise. Feet, ankles, calves, inner thighs and glutes all pulled together and contracted. Raise hips up and hold for 10–15 seconds. Repeat 3–5 times.

Tubing Side Step

Target Muscles:
Glutes, hips, feet, and core.
With glutes slightly back, navel up and in, keeping your toes square, step slowly side to side, keeping tension in the tubing. Hands on hips, chest up and shoulders back. Keep the upper body quiet (imagine balancing a cup of water on each shoulder). Remember to keep toes facing straight (forward).

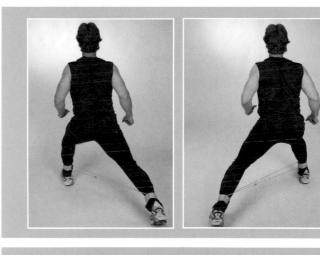

Tubing Backward Step

Target Muscles:
Glutes, hips, quadriceps, feet, and core.
Maintain ideal posture. Go forward in a skating motion. Repeat movement backwards. Excellent for strength in the hips and legs and improved balance.

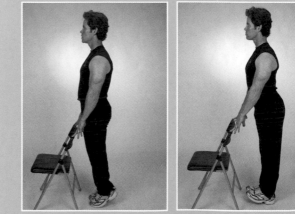

Calf/Shin Raise

Target Muscles:
Calf and shin muscles.
In ideal posture position, with the knees slightly bent, raise up on toes. Hold for 2–3 seconds at the top position. Alternate back and forth, raising heels up and toes up.

STRENGTH TRAINING

Upper Body

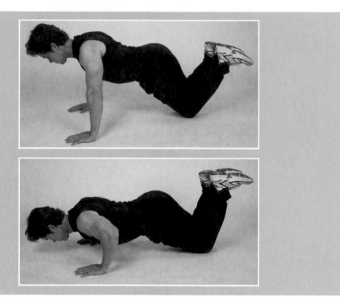

Modified Push-up

Target Muscles:
Chest, triceps, anterior deltoid, and core.

Start with knees together, toes off the floor, hips up, navel pulled up and in, and hands slightly wider than shoulder width. Keeping shoulder blades together, lower chest until elbows form a 90-degree angle. Keeping elbows out, hold, then push from chest to bring body back to start position. Exhale as you push up.

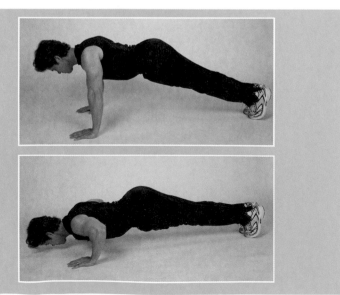

Push-up

Target Muscles:
Chest, triceps, anterior deltoid, and core.

With toes on the floor and hands wider than shoulder width apart, lower chest toward the floor, stopping when elbows reach a 90-degree angle. Keep shoulder blades back and down, maintain a neutral pelvis by squeezing glutes and pulling navel in. Keeping elbows out, hold, then push from chest to bring body back to start position.

Dumbbell Chest Press

Target Muscles:

Chest, triceps, and shoulders.
Keep knees bent and shoulder
blades together. Start with
weight above your shoulders.
Lower the weight slowly
keeping hands directly above
your elbows until they form a
90-degree angle from the
shoulder joint. (Do not let
elbows go below shoulders.)
As you push the weight up,
drive your elbows in, squeezing
your chest muscles.

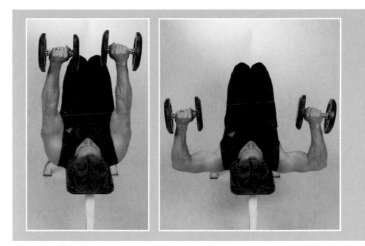

Dumbbell Chest Fly

Target Muscles:

Chest and anterior deltoid.
Keep knees bent and
shoulder blades together.
Lower the weight slowly,
keeping elbows slightly bent
until they are aligned with
the shoulder joint.

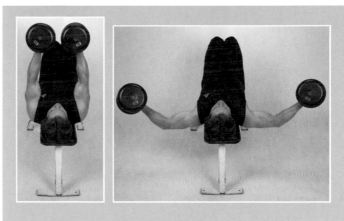

Dumbbell Row

Target Muscles:

*Latissimus, trapezius,
rhomboids, biceps, and core.*
Bend over with a flat back.
Bend knees, squeeze your
glutes, and pull navel in. Pull
shoulder blades back and
down, keeping a flat back.
While squeezing elbows tight
to the body, raise weight until
elbow reaches midline. Keep
shoulders even.

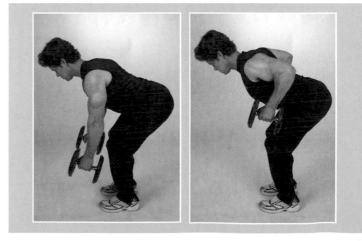

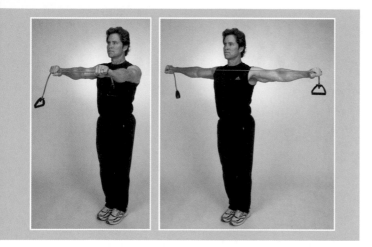

Tubing Wide Pull

Target Muscles:
Rear deltoids, trapezius, triceps, rhomboids, and core.
Maintain ideal posture position. Arms straight, shoulder blades down and back, pull tubing across chest until body forms a "T." Keep tension in tubing and wrists straight. Keep rib cage up and pull navel up and in. To increase intensity bring hands closer together to start or change color of tubing. (Great exercise to work those posture muscles.)

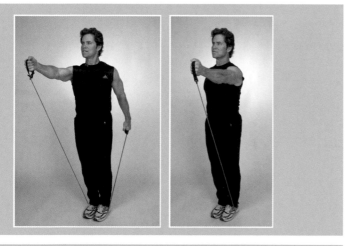

Tubing Straight Arm Raise

Target Muscles:
Anterior deltoid, biceps, and core.
Maintain ideal posture. Place tubing under the feet. Keep arms straight, thumb up, raise arm to chin height. Move with a cross-country skiing motion.

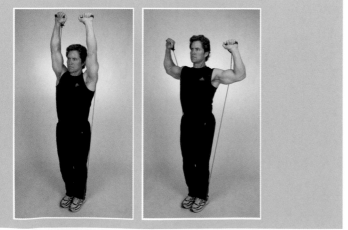

Tubing Shoulder Press

Target Muscles:
Anterior deltoid, triceps, and core.
Maintain ideal posture with tubing underneath feet and behind elbows. Extend arms overhead, chest up and shoulders back and down. Do not arch back, keep glutes tight and navel pulled up and in. Lower elbows until they align with shoulders. Keep hands directly over elbows. This exercise can be more demanding on the shoulder joint, so start slowly with very little resistance.

Tubing Lateral Raise

Target Muscles:

Medial deltoid, upper trapezius, and core.

Ideal posture position, place tubing under your feet and cross tubing. Elbows at your side in a 90-degree angle. Keeping your chest up and shoulders back and down, with the tubing handle in hands, raise elbow to shoulder height keeping arms at 90 degrees. At the top position, the hands, elbows and shoulders should be flat (imagine balancing a cup of water on each joint).

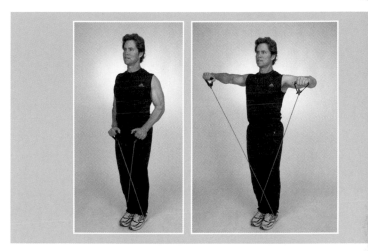

Biceps Curl

Target Muscles:

Biceps, forearms, upper back, and core.

Maintaining ideal posture, stand on the tubing or hold dumbbells with palms up. Keep elbows back, raise hands up to chest height only, and keep wrists firm. Squeeze biceps at the top and lower slowly. To increase the forearm muscle involvement, turn hand so the thumb is pointing up (hammer curls).

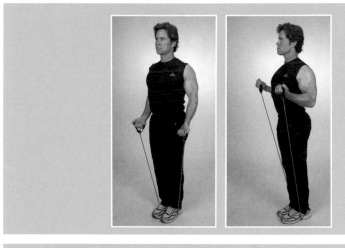

Triceps Kickbacks

Target Muscles:

Triceps, glutes, back, and core.

Grasping a dumbbell in each hand, lean upper body forward 45 degrees, flat back, shoulder blades together, glutes tight, navel pulled up and in, elbows anchored at your side. Straighten elbows and extend arms behind you in a slow and controlled movement. Shoulders, elbows, and wrists should be aligned at end of movement.

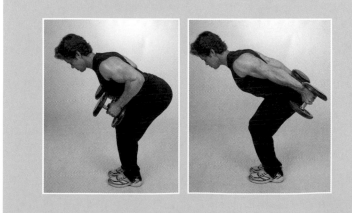

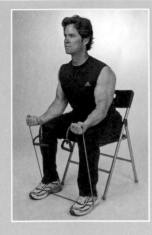

Wrist/Forearm

Target Muscles:
Wrist, hand, and forearm.
Seated position with ideal posture. Palms up, elbows touching thigh, handles in, flex forearms.

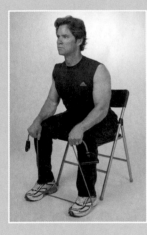

Seated position with ideal posture. Palms down, elbows touching thigh, handles out, extend forearms.

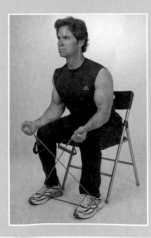

Seated position with ideal posture. Cross tubing, handles out, rotate forearms.

STRENGTH TRAINING

Core

Ab Crunch

Target Muscles:
Core.

Place your fingertips lightly on your thighs. Keep your glutes tight and pull navel up and in throughout the entire movement. Slowly lift your chest up, reaching your fingertips to your knees. Keep your eyes looking to the ceiling. Exhale during exertion (when coming up). Add rotation as you advance. Maintain adequate space between chest and chin.

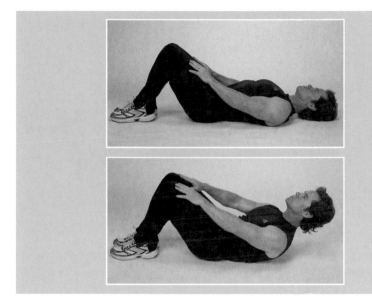

Hip Curl

Target Muscles:
Core.

Lying on your back, arms overhead, try to keep arms straight and shoulder blades down and in, knees together, heels close to your glutes. Pull navel up and in and slowly pull your knees into your chest. Do not lower knees past the hips. When you first begin, your range of motion may be small. As you get stronger this will slowly improve. A great exercise for core strength and lower back flexibility.

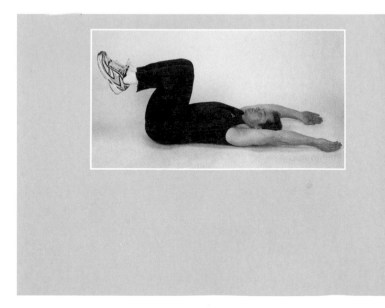

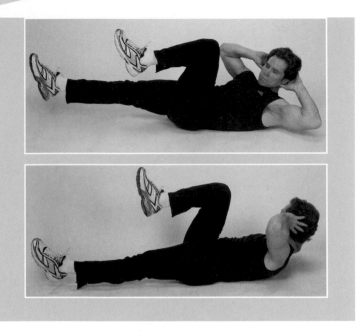

Bicycle

Target Muscles:
Core.

Lie on floor with shoulder blades retracted, navel pulled up and in, glutes tight. With both legs raised slightly off ground, bring one knee toward midline while bringing opposite elbow toward knee. Alternate knees. To make the exercise easier, keep the heel of the straightened leg touching the floor.

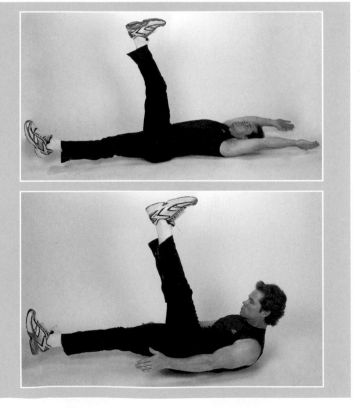

Scissor

Target Muscles:
Core.

Lie on floor with your arms overhead. As you bring one leg up, bring both arms forward and repeat with opposite leg. To make exercise easier, keep the heel of the straightened leg touching the floor.

Crunch Combination

Target Muscles:
Core.
Lie on the floor. Finger tips behind the ears. Knees bent, feet off the floor. Slowly bring chest up and pull knees in.

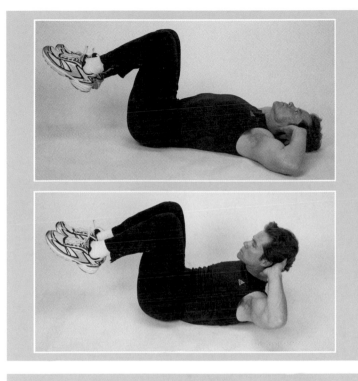

Seated Twist

Target Muscles:
Core.
Start in a seated position with knees bent. Lean back, keep rib cage up, navel pulled up and in, and feet touching the floor. Extend arms with hands apart, slowly twisting side to side while maintaining ideal posture.

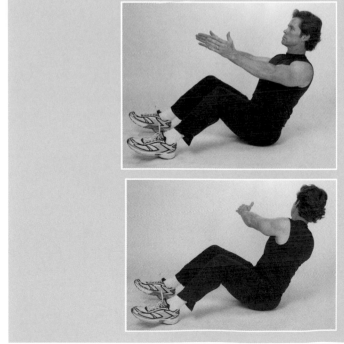

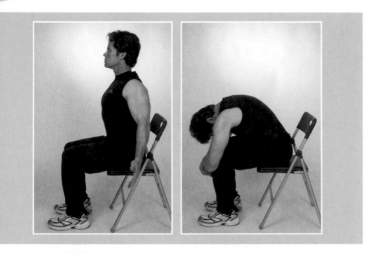

Chair Back Extension

Target Muscles:
Upper and lower back.
Sitting with ideal posture, tuck the chin, round the spine and pull your navel in. Repeat 4–10 times.

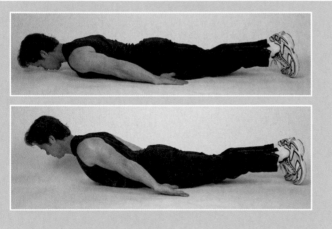

Prone Back Extension

Target Muscles:
Lower and upper back.
Lie face down, extend arms at your side, palms facing down, and legs straight. Contract glutes and pull navel up and in. Lift chest off the ground, keeping head in neutral position. Keep the chin pulled in gently. Hold movement for 5–10 seconds

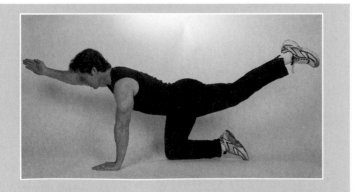

Spinal Balance

Target Muscles:
Back, core, shoulders, and glutes.
On hands and knees, extend one arm forward and lift the opposite leg backward until arm, leg, and core form a straight line. Contract glutes and pull navel up and in. Hold for 5–10 seconds. Repeat on opposite side.

Plank

Target Muscles:

Core, shoulders, and legs.
Position body with toes on floor, resting on elbows and hands. Hold body in straight alignment by tightening glutes and pull navel up and in. A great exercise for conditioning the entire core. Hold movement for 5–30 seconds.

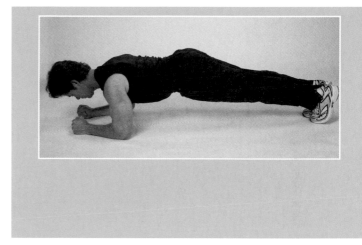

Advanced Plank

Target Muscles:

Core, shoulders, and legs.
Begin in plank position. Slowly raise one leg off floor, maintaining balance and tight glutes with navel pulled up and in. Keep hips square and hold movement. Alternate legs. Hold movement for 5–30 seconds.

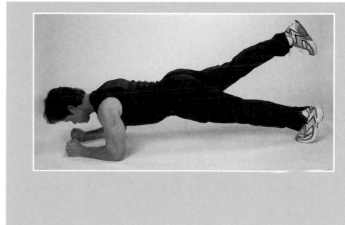

Modified Side Plank

Target Muscles:

Core, shoulders, and hips.
Place hand directly under shoulder. Place weight evenly between hand, knee, and foot. Raise hips high. Hold 5–30 seconds. Repeat on opposite side.

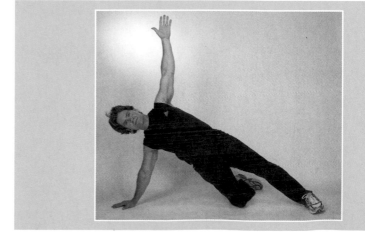

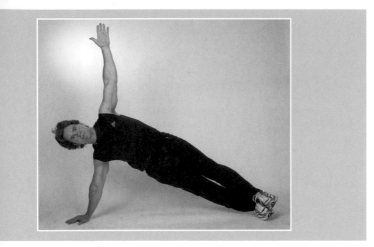

Side Plank

Target Muscles:
Core, shoulders, and hips.
Balance on hand and side of foot, hips high, maintain strong core, feet together. Raise hips high. Hold 5–30 seconds. Repeat on opposite side.

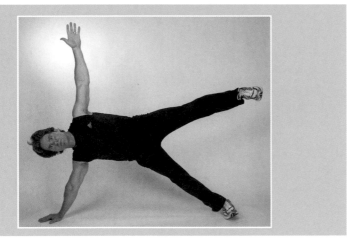

Advanced Side Plank

Target Muscles:
Core, shoulders, and hips.
From side plank position raise top leg. Raise hips high. Hold 5–30 seconds. Repeat on opposite side.

STRETCHING/FLEXIBILITY

The benefits of stretching are many, from decreasing stress to improving muscle imbalances. Stretching exercises should be performed after the body is warmed up or at the end of your exercise program. There are virtually hundreds of different stretching exercises to choose from. I have chosen very basic stretches that cover the entire body. Don't neglect the stretching portion of your exercise program. Start with just a few stretching exercises and gradually build from there. Focus on proper body alignment and breathing (deep, slow breathing). Stretching exercises may be done daily. A few general rules apply to stretching:

1. Hold each stretch for 10 to 60 seconds.
2. Maintain ideal posture throughout all stretches.
3. Do not stretch to a point of discomfort.

Big 3 Tubing Stretch

Target Muscles:
Hamstrings, adductors, hips, and lower back.

Lying on your back, place tubing or towel around your shoe. Keeping one leg straight and touching the floor, bring the other leg straight back, to your side and across the body. Maintain a slight bend in the knees for all 3 stretches. Do the same with the opposite leg. (3 stretches each leg)

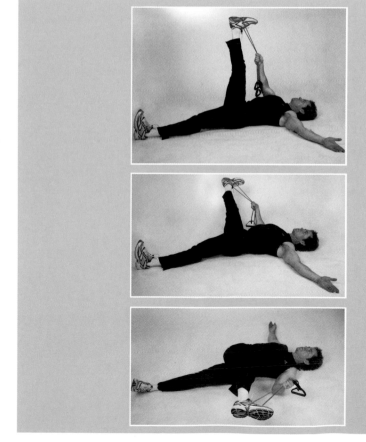

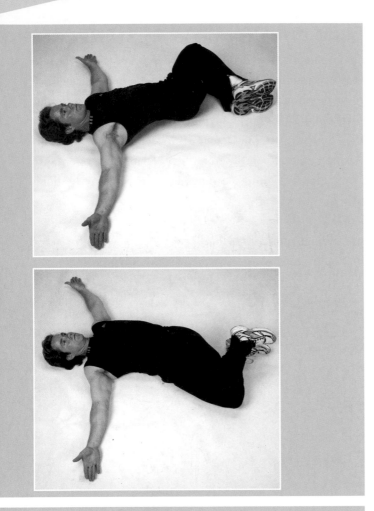

Golfer's Stretch

Target Muscles:
Hips, core, and lower back.
Lie on your back, arms out to the side, bend knees with thighs and knees together. Slowly rock knees side to side.

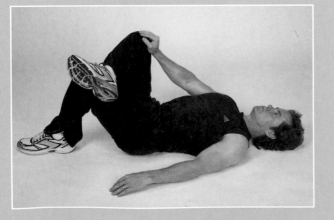

Piriformis 1 (Beginner)

Target Muscles:
Hips and piriformis.
On your back, cross knee. Gently push knee away from your upper body with your hand. To increase the intensity of this stretch, sit up with your back against a wall.

Piriformis 2 (Advanced)

Target Muscles:
Hips and piriformis.
On your back, cross knee. Gently pull knee into your opposite shoulder.

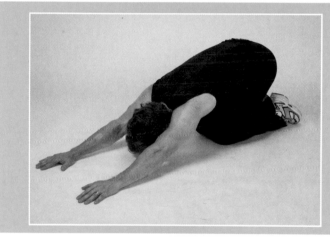

Child's Pose

Target Muscles:
Back, shoulders, and lats.
From hands and knees, push hips back toward the heels. Keep arms straight reaching forward. To stretch out your lats, reach to the side. A great relaxation stretch.

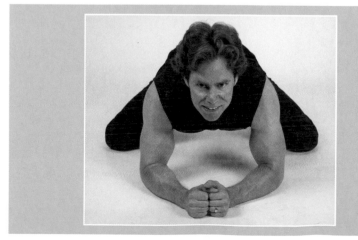

Frog Stretch

Target Muscles:
Adductors, hips, and back.
Resting on knees and forearms, spread legs apart, chest up, flat back. To increase stretch move hips slowly back.

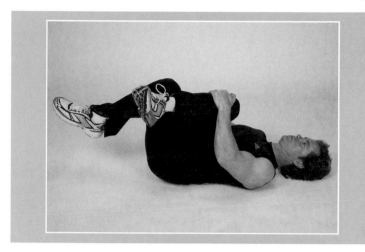

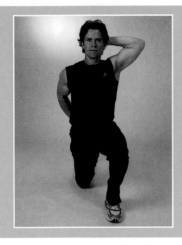

Kneeling Hip Flexor

Target Muscles:

Hip flexor and quadriceps.
On right knee, place right
hand on right glute. Place left
hand behind your head,
pull elbow back to open up
the rib cage. Contract glutes
and pull navel up and in.
Try to pull your right knee
forward (isometrically)
without changing your pelvic
tilt. Repeat on the opposite
side. A great stretch for
runners and golfers.

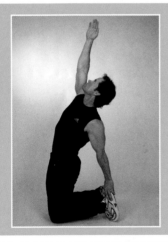

Modified Camel

Target Muscles:

Quadriceps, hip flexors,
shoulders, core, and neck.
From kneeling position, place
left hand on left heel and raise
right hand overhead. Squeeze
your glutes to protect your
lower back. As you reach up
and back with your right hand,
try to push the hips forward,
squeezing the glutes and
pulling your navel into
your spine.

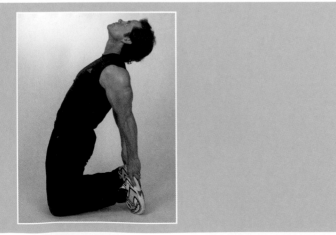

Camel

Target Muscles:

Quadriceps, hip flexors,
shoulders, core, and neck.
As you become comfortable
with the modified camel, try
this regular camel exercise.
From kneeling position, place
hands on heels. Gently press
the hips forward and lift the
chest to the sky. Tighten your
glutes and pull your navel into
your spine.

Advanced Hamstring Stretch

Target Muscles:
Hamstrings, glutes, back, and core.

Place hands on each side of the forward leg to support your posture, slight bend in forward leg, chest up, and maintain a flat back. Pull navel up and in. Straighten forward leg for 1 second and then bend forward leg and hold for 15–30 seconds. Repeat 2–3 times on each side.

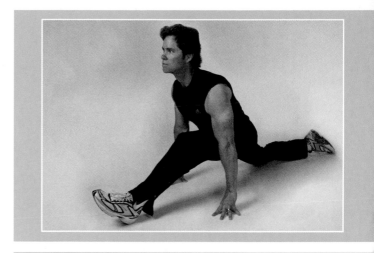

Cat and Dog

Target Muscles:
Back, core, shoulders, and neck.

On hands and knees, round your spine (cat position), pull your navel into your spine, in the dog position bring your head up, pull your shoulders back and down and change pelvic positions. In both movements, keep your arms slightly bent and knees bent at 90-degree angle.

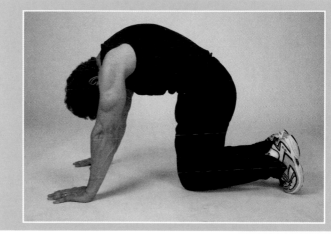

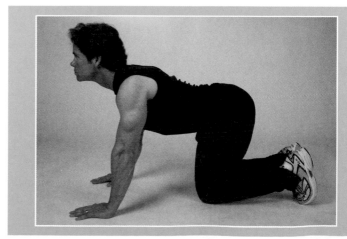

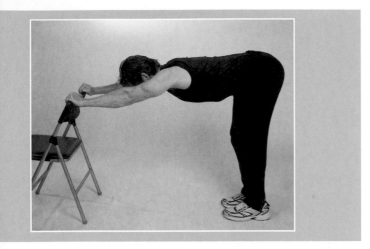

Standing Downward Dog

Target Muscles:
Full body.

Hold onto a fixed object, feet shoulder width apart. Push hips back and push shoulders toward floor. Keep back, head and arms in neutral alignment. Modify stretch by slightly bending knees. A great stretch that is easy to perform and can be done virtually anywhere.

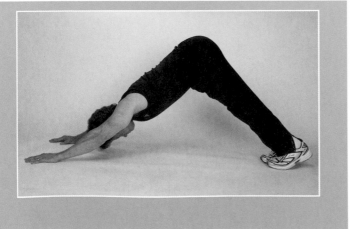

Standing Upward Dog

Target Muscles:
Full body.

Feet shoulder width apart, place hands on fixed object, face forward, chest up, glutes tight, pull navel up and in. Slowly pull hips forward, head back, shoulders down and in.

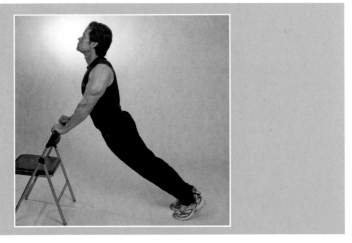

Downward Dog

Target Muscles:
Full body.

Hands slightly wider than shoulder width, fingers spread apart, wrists neutral (flat). Push hips toward ceiling and push chest toward your thighs, knees slightly bent. As you become warmed up, straighten legs more and slowly lower heels to the floor, pull navel up and in. Hold stretch 10–30 seconds, repeat 2–3 times.

Upward Dog

Target Muscles:
Full body.
Hands directly under shoulders, from the downward dog position, slowly lower your hips, pull toes underneath, squeeze your glutes, pull head up and shoulders back and down. In both movements, keep your arms slightly bent. Pull navel up and in. Keep knees slightly off the floor. Hold stretch 10–30 seconds, repeat 2–3 times.

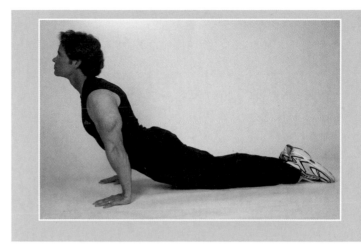

Modified Boat

Target Muscles:
Hip flexor, quads, shoulders, and back.
Grab ankle or top of foot. Straighten arm and leg, slowly raise bent knee slightly off the floor.

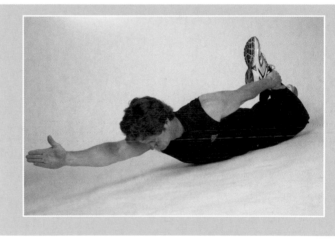

Boat

Target Muscles:
Hip flexor, quads, shoulders, and back.
Legs together, grab ankle or top of foot. Slowly raise knees slightly off the floor.

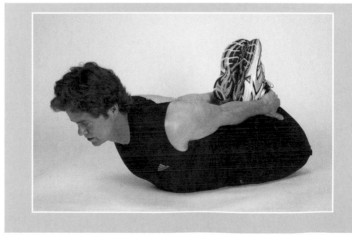

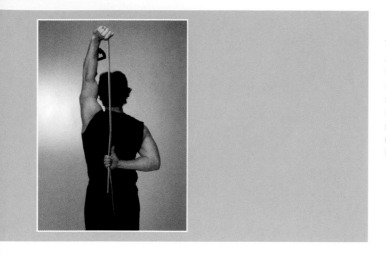

Rotator Cuff

Target Muscles:

Shoulders and rotator cuff.

Use a broomstick, towel, or rubber tubing. With arm straight overhead, grab implement with thumb up, slowly pull bent arm up while maintaining ideal posture. Don't force this stretch.

SAMPLE EXERCISE PROGRAMS

I have designed a few sample exercise routines for the beginner, intermediate, and advanced exerciser. The goal with all exercises is to challenge the body while maintaining ideal posture and good technique throughout each exercise. Start slowly and listen to your body.

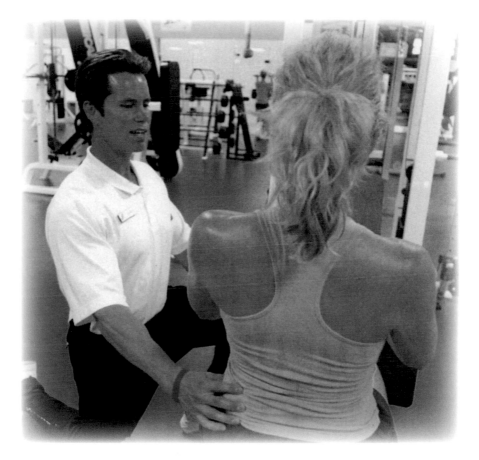

Beginner
Dynamic Warm-up: Spend a few minutes getting your body warmed up with dynamic stretches. Use slow and controlled movements. Get into a habit of warming up your body before you exercise. 2 minutes.
Foundational: Squat, lunge, half moon, thoracic extensions
Cardiovascular Exercise: 5–15 minutes, at an easy intensity level, 2–4 times per week. Maintain ideal posture throughout your cardiovascular exercise portion.
Strength Training: The exercises here cover the large muscle groups. Focus on perfect technique with 1–2 sets per exercise of 4–10 reps per set, 2–3 times per week.

Recommended Exercises	Page
Squats	252
Tubing side steps	261
Tubing wide pull	264
Back extension	270
Modified pushup	262

Stretching: Standing up-and-down dog

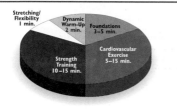

Beginning
exercise program
twenty to forty minutes
two or three times per week

Intermediate	
Posture	
Dynamic Warm-up: 2–3 minutes.	
Foundational: Squat, lunge, warrior 1 and 2, half moon, thoracic extensions. 5 minutes.	
Cardiovascular Exercise: 15–20 minutes, 2–4 times per week. Start adding in interval training (higher-intensity bursts between recovery periods). Maintain ideal posture throughout your cardiovascular exercise session.	
Strength Training: 2–3 sets per exercise, 8–12 reps per set, 2–3 times per week. You may want to split up your strength training routine (upper body Monday and Thursday, lower body Tuesday and Friday). Maintain ideal posture and technique with each exercise. 15–30 minutes.	
Recommended Exercises	**Page**
Lower Body:	
Squats: Hold each exercise for 3–5 seconds at the bottom of the movement, maintaining perfect alignment.	252
Step-ups: 8–10 reps per set, hold each exercise for 2–5 seconds at the top of the movement.	258
Tubing side steps: Ideal posture, use green tubing, go slow and feel the hips and legs working.	261
Upper Body:	
Modified –or– regular pushups	262
Dumbbell rows	263
Thoracic extensions: No weight, hold movement at the top	256
Standing biceps curls	
Core:	
Back extension (prone position)	270
Spinal balance	270
Stretching: Downward and upward dog, hip stretch. 2–3 minutes	278–279

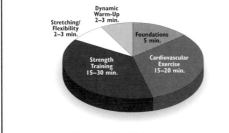

Dynamic Warm-Up 2–3 min.
Stretching/ Flexibility 2–3 min.
Foundations 5 min.
Strength Training 15–30 min.
Cardiovascular Exercise 15–20 min.

Intermediate
exercise program
sixty to seventy minutes
two to four times per week

I have split the advanced routine into two different workouts. Each workout may be completed one or two times per week. Remember to incorporate rest and recovery into your weekly program.

Advanced	
Workout #1: Monday/Thursday	
Posture	
Dynamic Warm-up: 2–3 minutes.	
Foundational: Squat, lunge, warrior 3, warrior 1 & 2, spread eagle, dancer, T-extensions, half moon, standing upward and downward dog. 5–7 minutes.	
Cardiovascular Exercise: 15–30 minutes of steady-state (maintaining the same intensity) exercise, moderate to high intensity.	
Strength Training: 20–30 minutes.	
Recommended Exercises	**Page**
Lower Body:	
Squat: 3 or 4 sets, 8–12 reps per set	258
Straight leg lunge: 3 sets; hold each exercise for 20–30 seconds. Don't forget to breathe.	259
Step-ups: 3 or 4 sets, 8–12 reps; hold each exercise for 1–2 seconds at the top of the movement.	258
Tubing side step: Maintain ideal posture. Use green or red tubing.	261
Calf/shin raise: 3 sets of 8–12 reps; hold exercise for 1–2 seconds at the top of the movement. Maintain ideal posture.	261
Hip extensions or kneeling hamstring	260
Core:	
Side plank: Hold movement for 15–30 seconds.	272
Seated twist	269
Hip curl: 6–10 reps, slowly.	267
Stretching: Hold each movement for 10–30 seconds, repeat 2 times.	
Recommended Exercises	**Page**
Downward and upward dog	278–279
Kneeling hip flexes	276

Stretching/Flexibility 2 min. · Dynamic Warm-Up 2–3 min. · Foundations 5–7 min. · Cardiovascular Exercise 15–30 min. · Strength Training 20–30 min.

Advanced
exercise program
sixty-five to seventy-five minutes
once or twice per week

Advanced
Workout #2: Tuesday/Friday

Posture

Dynamic Warm-up: 2–3 minutes.

Foundational: Squat, lunge, warrior 3, warrior 1 and 2, spread eagle, dancer, T-extensions, half moon, standing upward and downward dog. 5–7 minutes.

Cardiovascular Exercise: 15–25 minutes of interval training, moderate to high intensity.

Strength Training: 20–30 minutes.

Recommended Exercises	Page
Upper Body:	
Pushup	262
Dumbbell chest press	263
Dumbbell row	263
Tubing wide pull	264
Lateral raise (tubing or dumbbells)	265
Thoracic extension	256
Biceps curl	265
Triceps kickbacks	265
Core:	
Plank: Hold movement for 15–30 seconds.	271
Bicycle/scissor	268
Seated twist	269

Stretching: Downward and upward dog, piriformis 1. Hold each movement for 10–30 seconds, repeat 2 times.

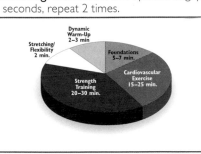

Advanced
exercise program
sixty-five to seventy-five minutes
once or twice per week

EXERCISE LOG

WEEK OF ____/____/____

	Dynamic Warm-up 2–3 min.	Foundations 5–7 min.	Cardiovascular 15–30 min.	Strength 10–40 min.	Flexibility 1–5 min.	Daily physical activity	Comments
Monday	3 min.	5 min.	Elliptical training (high intensity) 15	Lower body Core 35			Worked on posture with all exercises
Tuesday	2 min.	3 min.	Treadmill walking (moderate intensity) 20	Chest Back 30		15 min. walk after dinner	Focused on techniques and strength training
Wednesday	before yoga class			Shoulders Arms Core 30		Power yoga class 60 min.	Breathing significantly better Great class!
Thursday	2 min.	7 min.	Stair climbers (high intensity) 15				High energy Felt strong
Friday	2 min.	6 min.	Stationary bike (moderate intensity) 20	Lower body Core 35			Working on better alignment and lower body
Saturday	3 min.	7 min.	Played tennis 90				Backhand needs work!
Sunday	5 min. before golf	5 min.				Walked 18 holes of golf	Felt great after walking the 18

Appendix C
ON TARGET LIVING
DAILY LOGS

Use the logs contained in this appendix to develop and reinforce your new healthy nutrition and exercise routines. Remember, start slowly and make small changes.

A friend is a present you give yourself.

—Robert Louis Stevenson

On Target Living is a guide for living a life in balance, with energy and vitality. Meeting our basic hierarchy of needs— nutrition, exercise, rest, and rejuvenation—enhances our lives. On Target Living can help us meet these needs, one small step at a time.

—Chris Johnson
speaker/author

On Target Living—**FOOD TARGET**

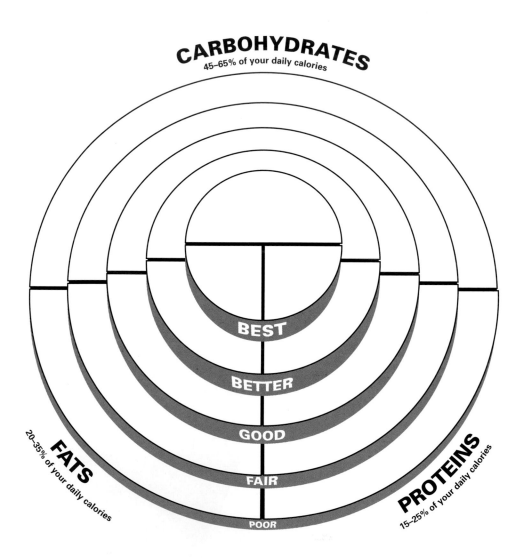

On Target Living—**DAILY FOOD LOG**

DAILY FOOD LOG		

Day: _____ Date: _____

MEAL	DESCRIPTION	TARGET
Breakfast Time: _____		CARBOHYDRATES FATS PROTEINS
Snack 1 Time: _____		CARBOHYDRATES FATS PROTEINS
Lunch Time: _____		CARBOHYDRATES FATS PROTEINS
Snack 2 Time: _____		CARBOHYDRATES FATS PROTEINS
Dinner Time: _____		CARBOHYDRATES FATS PROTEINS
Snack 3 Time: _____		CARBOHYDRATES FATS PROTEINS

Water (8 oz.)	☐ ☐ ☐ ☐ ☐ ☐ ☐ ☐ ☐ ☐ ☐
Sleep (hours)	4 ☐　5 ☐　6 ☐　7 ☐　8 ☐　9 ☐　10 ☐
Activity/exercise	☐ Dynamic ☐ Foundations ☐ Cardio ☐ Strength ☐ Flexibility ☐ Other
Breathing breaks	☐ ☐ ☐ ☐ ☐ ☐ ☐ ☐ ☐ ☐
Meditation/napping	☐ ☐ ☐ ☐ ☐ ☐ ☐ ☐ ☐ ☐ ☐
Comments	

On Target Living—**EXERCISE LOG**

EXERCISE LOG
WEEK OF ___/___/___

	Dynamic Warm-up 2–3 min..	Foundations 5–7 min.	Cardiovascular 15–30 min	Strength 10–40 min.	Flexibility 1–5 min.	Daily physical activity	Comments
Monday							
Tuesday							
Wednesday							
Thursday							
Friday							
Saturday							
Sunday							

INDEX

A

Acid levels, 20, 34–41, 93, 125, 130–131

Acid reflux, 12, 34, 35, 36, 38, 53, 54, 102, 120, 221

Acidic, 20, 34–41, 93, 120, 124–127, 129, 132

Acidosis, 129–130

Adrenal glands, 48, 124

Adrenaline, 38, 130

Aerobic, 204, 206–207

Agave nectar, 40, 77, 78, 80, 151

Alcohol, 35, 36, 40, 50, 119, 124, 125, 127, 130, 151, 166, 184

Alkaline, 34–41, 79, 87, 120–121, 122, 125, 127, 129, 131, 132, 218, 221

Allergies, 54, 121, 133

Almond butter, 103, 117, 135, 142, 154, 167, 190, 191, 227

Almond milk, 39, 40, 60, 86, 121, 154, 189, 219

Almond oil, 40, 103, 117, 154, 167, 221. **In recipes: 230, 243**

Almonds, 39, 40, 60, 70, 74, 82, 83, 87, 103, 114, 117, 128, 130, 146, 154, 160, 164, 167, 168, 171, 188, 189, 218, 221. **In recipes: 227, 228, 230, 233**

Alzheimer's disease, 114

Amino acids, 81–83, 87, 94

Anaerobic, 204, 206, 207

Animal fats, 43, 44, 83, 97, 101, 112

Anterior deltoid, 262, 263, 264

Antibiotics, 38, 43, 44, 45, 84, 88, 130, 152

Antidepressants, 15

Antioxidants, 13, 19, 20, 22, 66, 68, 101, 102, 121, 122, 124, 127, 218, 221, 222

Anxiety, 15, 26, 177

Arachidonic acid, 112, 113, 131

Arachidonic overload, 113, 131

Artery walls, 106

Artesian water, 40, 126, 155, 218, 220

Arthritis, 54, 97, 99, 105, 113, 114, 124

Artificial sweeteners, 35, 39, 40, 77, 119, 130, 131, 150–151, 152

Aspirin, 54, 55, 106, 114

Attention Deficit Hyperactivity Disorder (ADHD), 99, 108, 133

Avocados, 40, 74, 103, 114, 117, 153, 155, 167, 221. **In recipes: 232**

B

Baked goods, 26, 66, 68, 74, 76, 77, 100, 102, 117, 175, 177, 187, 244

Bananas, 40, 67, 71, 74, 87, 89, 146, 153, 166, 173, 219. **In recipes: 231**

Barley, 40, 69, 71, 130, 154

Barley grass, 40, 122, 130, 153, 158, 221, 222

Beats per minute (bpm), 206

Beef tenderloin, 154

Beer, 35, 39, 40, 119, 124, 130, 131

Behavior change, 138, 139, 142, 143, 179–181, 198

Beverages, 13, 21, 30, 31, 32, 34–37, 39, 40, 41, 43, 44, 45, 56, 61, 64, 66, 69, 86, 88, 89, 100, 108, 109, 119–127, 130, 131, 132, 133, 135, 140, 141, 145, 147, 150, 151, 152, 153, 158, 159, 160, 162, 163, 168, 221–222

Biking, 162, 201, 203, 204, 205, 224, 247, 251

Bionic woman, 192–193

Black currant oils, 113

Black hole, 75–76, 80

Bleached, 103

Blender, 141, 173, 230, 231, 238, 245

Blood clotting, 106

Blood glucose, 15, 24, 26, 30, 31, 32, 53, 66, 67, 68, 69, 71, 72, 73–75, 76, 77, 80, 82, 83, 100, 106, 123, 148, 151, 156, 204, 218, 221, 222

Blood pH, 34–36, 129

Blood pressure, 10, 27, 48, 50, 52, 54, 55, 90, 95, 99, 100, 106, 107, 124, 125, 193, 194, 204, 212, 221

Blueberries, 35, 37, 40, 67, 70, 146, 153

Body cleansing, 124

Body fat, 18, 19, 20, 24, 25, 37, 44, 72, 162, 163, 194, 219

Bone density, 129, 207, 258

Bone loss, 205

Bone regeneration, 129

Borage oil, 117, 221

Brain power, 19–20, 22, 67, 68, 77, 83, 84, 94, 99, 108, 221

Breads, 18, 68, 70, 71, 73, 74, 76, 77, 81, 82, 87, 92, 110, 134, 135, 142, 146, 147, 154, 158, 160, 161, 166, 170, 171, 187, 189, 190, 191, 219. *See also* white bread, whole-grain bread.

Breathing, 35, 39, 40, 50, 51, 131, 140, 144, 179, 180, 181, 206, 209, 210, 212, 218, 222, 223, 273

Broccoli, 17, 26, 40, 60, 66, 68, 71, 70, 74, 80, 87, 130, 140, 141, 153, 166, 218, 219, 220. **In recipes:** 229, 233

Broccoli slaw, 70, 153, 219. **In recipes:** 233

Brown fat, 99, 112–113

Buffalo, 55, 86, 92, 154, 167, 189. **In recipes:** 239

Buffering elements, 20, 35, 36, 41, 93, 125, 129, 130

Building blocks, 47–50, 108, 218, 221

Butter vs. Margarine, 117, 162

C

C-pap, 54

Caffeine, 35, 50, 76, 119, 121, 124, 131

Cakes, 26, 74, 77, 100, 102, 117, 175, 187. **In recipes:** 244

Calcium, 35, 36, 37, 60, 79, 93, 125, 128, 130–131, 132

Calf, 261, 284

Cancer, 27, 68, 69, 80, 96, 97, 99, 101, 102, 109, 110, 113, 114, 121, 123, 125, 132

Candida, 78, 88

Capric acid, 102

Caprylic acid, 102, 121

Carbohydrates, 8, 17, 18, 19, 20, 22, 26, 28, 29, 60, 61, 64, 65, 66–80, 82, 87, 89, 90, 91, 94, 100, 101, 148, 151, 153, 160, 163, 166, 167, 169–174, 175, 180, 218, 220

Carbon atoms, 103

Cardiovascular exercise, 15, 195, 197, 199, 200, 201, 202, 204–207, 210, 213, 222, 281, 282, 283, 284, 285

Cardiovascular system, 35, 99, 106, 202

Cashews, 103, 117

Cell, 17, 20, 24, 26, 27, 30–33, 72, 81, 82, 94, 96, 99, 100, 101, 103, 106–107, 110, 112, 121, 123, 134, 162, 175, 181

Cell membrane, 27, 31–32, 33, 99, 100, 103, 106, 107, 134

Cellular health, 30–31, 33, 54–55, 72, 95, 99, 106, 144, 158, 181, 218, 221

Central nervous system, 66, 106, 202, 207, 247, 258

Cheeses, 18, 19, 39, 40, 86, 96, 110, 114, 117, 130, 133, 134, 154, 160, 167, 189. **In recipes:** 229, 230, 234, 238, 240, 242

Chest press, 209, 263, 285

Chicken, 26, 40, 55, 70, 74, 84, 86, 92, 95, 142, 154, 161, 162, 167, 169, 170, 186. **In recipes:** 232, 235, 238, 240

Chips, 24, 68, 75, 89, 98, 100, 114, 119, 123, 134, 147, 148, 154, 175, 177, 178–179, 184

Choline, 84, 124, 134

Coconut, 37, 40, 101, 102, 117

Cod, 85, 154, 167

Cod liver oil, 30, 39, 40, 55, 83, 105, 111, 112, 114, 117, 130, 135, 140, 146, 154, 159, 160, 167, 180, 188, 189, 190, 191, 193, 198, 218, 219, 221. **In recipes:** 227

Coffee, 18, 34, 35, 36, 39, 40, 76, 120, 121, 125, 127, 130, 131, 160, 170

Cognitive skills, 83, 99

Colas, 39. *See* soda pop.

Conversions, 20, 105, 110, 113, 166

Cooking, 56, 70, 78, 102, 103, 104, 109, 110, 113, 114, 117, 130, 221, 227–245

Cooler, 141

Corn, 40, 71, 74, 81, 115, 153, 166, 172. **In recipes:** 229, 232, 233

Cortisol, 38, 48, 130, 163, 205

Cottonseed oil, 96, 112, 113, 115, 117

Crackers, 24, 68, 75, 100, 102, 114, 123, 134, 135, 142, 154, 184

Crete, 96–97

D

Daily food log, 32, 75, 104, 144–146, 164, 177, 178, 179, 219–220, 287–289

Dairy products, 17, 37, 39, 40, 43, 44, 60, 73, 74, 81, 83, 86–87, 88, 92, 96, 101, 102, 117, 121, 128, 130, 135, 154, 158, 160, 162, 167, 170, 172, 186, 218. **In recipes:** 227, 228, 234, 239, 244

Degummed, 103

Dehydration, 70, 124–125, 126, 127

Delayed onset muscle soreness, 213

Dementia, 97, 108

Deodorized, 103

Depression, 15, 37, 49, 97, 99, 108, 110, 112, 132, 180

Dextrose, 150

Diabetes, 10, 12, 24, 27, 32, 35, 95, 97, 99, 106–107, 110, 112, 113, 114, 120, 123, 125, 133, 193, 195, 201

Diet, 10, 12–14, 16–29, 30, 32, 34–42, 43–45, 50–51, 53–57, 59–62, 64–127, 130, 133–136, 140–142, 148–149, 151–152, 158–183, 186–191, 215–222, 223

Dieting, 7, 10, 14, 15, 16–22, 23, 27, 30, 32, 52, 54, 67, 72, 91, 158, 176–178, 179

Digestion, 35, 38, 49, 68–69, 71–72, 86–87, 88, 93, 100, 102, 121, 124, 127, 221

Doughnuts, 66, 68, 74, 100, 117, 177

Dumbbells, 211, 263, 265, 283, 285

Duration, 206

Dynamic stretching, 247–250

Dynamic stretching exercises, 247–250

E

Egg albumin, 88

Eggs, 19, 41, 43, 44, 54, 74, 81, 83, 84–85, 87, 88, 92, 101, 102, 104, 117, 130, 141, 142, 154, 160, 167, 190, 191, 218. **In recipes:** 229, 230, 231, 239, 240, 243, 244, 245

Eicosapentaenoic acid (EPA), 105, 110, 111, 112, 113

80/20 rule, 21–22, 199

Emotional Intelligence, 194

Energy bars, 90–91, 134, 142, 184

Essential amino acids, 81, 82, 83, 87, 94

Essential fatty acids, 27, 85, 96–97, 98, 99, 100, 102, 104–115, 116, 117, 121, 149, 150, 167, 221

Evening primrose oil, 40, 55, 113, 114, 115, 117, 150, 167, 219, 221

Exchange diet, 17, 22

Exercise, 7, 8, 12, 13, 14, 16, 20, 25, 27, 31, 32, 36, 37, 38, 41, 42, 47, 49, 50, 51, 52, 53, 58, 59, 91, 107, 127, 129, 131, 132, 140, 144, 162, 165, 175, 176, 178, 179, 181, 183, 185, 192–214, 215, 217, 218, 219, 222, 223, 224, 225, 226, 246–287, 290

Exercise routines, 211, 246, 281–285

Exercise tubing, 201, 208, 210–211, 261, 264, 265, 266, 273, 280, 282, 283, 284, 285

Extra-virgin coconut oil, 40, 55, 85, 101–102, 103, 113, 114, 117, 135, 140, 146, 150, 154, 158, 167, 190, 191, 193, 219, 221, 222. **In recipes:** 228, 244

Extra-virgin olive oil, 17, 26, 39, 40, 55, 95, 103, 114, 117, 134, 135, 140, 141, 146, 148, 149, 150, 154, 161, 162, 167, 169, 171, 172, 186, 187, 188, 190, 218, 219, 221, 227. **In recipes:** 229, 230, 232, 233, 234, 235, 236, 237, 238, 239, 240, 241, 242

F

Fast Food Nation, 97

Fast foods, 12–13, 40, 54, 58, 89, 97, 115, 123, 134, 161, 186

Fat categories, 100–115

Fat exchange, 17

Fat storing, 26, 72, 156, 157, 163, 172, 218

Fatigue, 10, 35, 42, 124, 132, 133

Feta, 117, 154, 167. **In recipes:** 242

Fiber, 13, 19, 22, 26, 66, 67, 68–70, 71, 73, 74, 80, 87, 92, 101, 109, 110, 147, 170, 171, 218, 220

Filberts, 110

Fish, 17, 37, 40, 54, 60, 70, 74, 81, 82, 85, 92, 97, 104, 105, 110, 111, 117, 128, 130, 141, 146, 154, 155, 167, 169, 171, 184–185, 186, 187, 188, 189, 190, 218, 221, 233, 240

Fish oils, 15, 30, 31, 39, 40, 55, 83, 104, 105, 106, 108, 110–112, 114, 115, 117, 130, 135, 140, 146, 154, 159, 160, 167, 180, 188, 189, 190, 191, 193, 198, 218, 219, 221, 227

Flank steak, 154, 167, 172

Flax meal, 54, 70, 89, 105, 106, 109, 110, 113, 114, 115, 117, 135, 154, 167, 189, 218, 221. **In recipes:** 231, 244

Flaxseed oil, 40, 55, 70, 83, 95, 104, 105, 108, 109–110, 111, 112, 113, 114, 115, 117, 135, 140, 146, 150, 154, 160, 167, 173, 188, 190, 193, 218, 221. **In recipes:** 227, 231

Flaxseeds, 15, 39, 70, 97, 104, 109, 110, 154, 155. **In recipes:** 228, 231, 243, 244

Flexibility, 129, 198, 201, 202, 203, 209–210, 213, 219, 222, 251, 256, 267, 273–280, 286, 289, 290

Flounder, 111

Folic acid, 84

Food and Drug Administration (FDA), 100–101, 148, 149

Food combinations, 25, 26, 64, 81–82, 145, 169–174

Food labels, 43, 55, 90, 95, 100–101, 147–152, 160

Food log, *see* Daily food log.

Food preparation, 140–143, 176, 181, 188, 227–245

Food pyramid, *see* USDA Food Pyramid.

Food quality, 8, 12–13, 15, 17, 18, 19, 21, 22, 24, 26–27, 28, 30–31, 32, 33, 39, 43–45, 50, 60, 61, 64, 66–68, 69, 70, 75, 77, 79, 80, 81, 82, 83, 84, 85, 86, 87, 88, 89, 90, 91, 92, 93, 94, 95, 97, 101, 102, 103, 104, 113, 114, 115, 116, 119, 120, 122, 125, 126, 132, 134, 144, 145, 147, 148, 152, 158–168, 170–173, 174, 176, 188, 218, 219, 221

Food steamer, 141

Food Target, 15, 20, 21, 51, 52, 54, 59–62, 64, 67, 75, 76, 77, 79, 80, 82, 87, 91, 93, 98, 116, 135, 144, 145, 168, 179, 181, 188, 215, 216, 217, 218, 219, 220, 221, 222, 288

Foundation exercises, 201, 202, 203, 210, 218, 222, 251–257, 282, 283, 284, 285

Fountain of youth, 50, 192–214

Fractionated oils, 91, 117, 149, 150

Free weights, 201, 208

Frequency of meals, *see* three-hour rule.

Fried foods, 35, 39, 40, 130, 131

Fructose, 73

Fruits, 12, 17, 19, 20, 21, 26, 32, 37, 39, 40, 44, 53, 59, 67, 68, 69, 70, 71, 73, 74, 85, 88, 97, 101, 121, 122, 131, 134, 135, 138, 140, 141, 142, 147, 153, 156, 162, 166, 184, 188, 189, 218, 220.
In recipes: 227, 228, 230, 231

Fruit juices, 13, 18, 69, 71, 73, 74, 110, 114, 122, 125, 126, 134, 141, 153–154, 161, 162, 184, 219, 222.
In recipes: 230, 234, 240

G

Galactose, 73

Gamma-linolenic acid (GLA), 112, 113

Gandhi, Mahatma, 109

Genetic factors, 25, 32, 33

Ghrelin, 49

Glucagon, 71, 72, 82–83

Glucose, 71, 72, 73, 74. *See* blood glucose.

Glutes, 200, 246, 252, 253, 254, 255, 256, 257, 258, 259, 260, 261, 262, 263, 264, 265, 267, 268, 270, 271, 276, 277, 278, 279

Glycemic Index, 67, 73–75

Goat, 86, 87, 167

Goat cheese, 40, 117

Goat milk, 37, 40, 60, 86–87, 88, 121, 154

Goatein, 88, 154

Gorgers, 23, 24

Gravity, 199, 200

Green tea, 39, 40, 120–121, 127, 131, 138, 160, 221, 222

Greenland Eskimos, 105

Growth hormones, 38, 43, 44, 84, 204, 205, 207

Gym on the Go, 211

H

Haddock, 111

Halibut, 85

Hamburger, 19, 86, 92, 161, 186

Hamstrings, 210, 252, 253, 254, 256, 258, 259, 260, 273, 277, 284

Hazelnut milk, 82, 86, 121

Hazelnuts, 82, 103, 154

HDL, 42, 54, 100, 103, 221

Healthy lifestyle, 16, 17, 32, 40, 51, 53, 54–56, 58, 107, 138, 139, 145, 174, 181, 187, 196, 199, 215, 217, 223–226

Healthy shopping, 153–155

Healthy snacks, 18, 24, 55, 88–89, 90, 103, 114, 134, 135, 136, 146, 164, 169, 170, 173, 174, 181, 185, 186, 188, 189, 190, 191, 212.
In recipes: 228, 230–231

Heart disease, 10, 27, 48–49, 58, 84, 96, 97, 101, 102, 103, 105, 110, 113, 114, 121, 122–123, 125

Heart rate, 50, 124, 206–207

Hemp, 87, 89, 117, 154, 167, 173.
In recipes: 230, 231

Hemp oil, 110

Herbal tea, 131

Hexane, 88

High-carbohydrate diet, 18, 22

High energy, 82, 187, 286

High-fructose corn syrup, 35, 55, 91, 119, 122–123, 148, 150, 152

High-oleic safflower oil, 103, 117, 154

High-protein diet, 19–20, 22, 67, 129

Hip flexor, 210, 276, 279

Hip fracture rates, 128

Hormonal imbalance, 18, 162

Hormones, 24, 31, 38, 43, 44, 48, 49, 71–72, 76, 81, 82–83, 84, 96, 100, 123, 130, 162, 163, 204, 205, 207, 258

Hot dogs, 17, 40, 134

Hunger hormone, 72, 76, 123

Hydrogenated oils, 101, 134, 149, 152, 167

Hydrogenation, 98

I

Ibuprofen, 114

Immune, 49, 81, 88, 99, 106, 121, 125, 205, 218, 221

Inflammation, 33, 35, 49, 95, 96, 97, 99, 100, 107–108, 112, 113, 114, 120, 122–123, 221

Inositol, 124

Insulin, 24, 26, 31–32, 54, 69, 71–72, 75, 76, 82, 99, 106–107, 123, 162, 163, 172

Insulin overshoot, 75

Intensity, 195, 197, 199, 204, 205, 206–207, 208, 209, 264, 265, 281, 282, 283, 284

Iodine, 35, 37, 39, 93, 125

Iron, 79, 86, 87, 221

Irritable bowel syndrome, 12, 35, 38, 102

J

Juice, 13, 69, 71, 73, 74, 78, 122, 134, 138, 141, 153–154, 162, 222

Juicer, 141

K

Kale, 37, 40, 54, 70, 71, 130, 146, 153, 166.
In recipes: 236

Ketone bodies, 20

Kidney beans, 40, 87, 154

Kidneys, 35, 41, 93, 124, 125

L

L-Carnitine, 124

Lauric acid, 102

LDL, 42, 100, 103, 221

Leafy green vegetables, 37, 60, 68, 69, 70, 71, 74, 97, 110, 112, 113, 114, 115, 130, 218, 220, 221

Lean muscle tissue, 25, 162, 163, 168, 188

Lecithin, 84

Legumes, 19, 40, 68, 71, 154, 166, 220

Leptin, 49, 123

Lignans, 109, 110

Linoleic acid (LA), 112, 113

Lipoprotein lipase, 23–24, 156, 157

Liver, 73, 93

Losing weight, *see* weight loss.

Low back pain, 124

Lower back, 267, 270, 273, 274, 276

M

Macadamia nut oil, 103, 117, 154, 221

Macadamia nuts, 103, 117

Mackerel, 85, 105, 110, 111

Macronutrients, 28, 61, 64–65, 87, 145, 151, 169–174

Magnesium, 35, 87, 93, 125, 130

Margarine, 17, 96, 100, 117, 150, 162, 167, 170

Marine oils, *see* fish oils.

Maslow's Hierarchy, 46–51

Meat, 18, 40, 43, 44, 81, 86, 96, 101, 104, 112, 113, 117, 154, 158, 161, 167, 218

Meditation, 131

Memory, 83, 108, 125

Metabolic rate, 24, 25, 96, 106, 156

Metabolism, 32, 37, 82–83, 93, 99, 106, 112, 123, 124, 156–157, 162, 206, 207, 218, 222, 258

Metal catalyst, 98

Microwave popcorn, 100, 117

Milk protein isolates, 87, 88

Mindful eating, 175–183

Mineral water, 39, 40, 120, 122, 125–126, 131, 138, 140, 142, 158, 193, 218, 220, 222

Minerals, 13, 19, 20, 22, 26, 35–36, 37, 39, 41, 66, 67, 68, 74, 78, 79, 101, 122–123, 124, 125, 126, 129–130, 171, 218, 220, 221, 222. *See also individual minerals.*

Monosodium glutamate (MSG), 40, 148

Monounsaturated fats, 27, 100, 102–104, 113, 115, 116, 149, 167, 221. *See also* omega-9.

Mood levels, 26, 50, 64, 76–77, 160, 194, 204, 217, 220

Motivation, 51, 139, 183, 194, 215, 217

Mozzarella, 154, 167. **In recipes:** 240

Muscle imbalances, 200, 209, 273

MyPyramid, *see* USDA Food Pyramid.

N

National Cancer Institute, 69, 80

Natural Bodybuilding, 199

Natural peanut butter, 74, 81, 87, 92, 103, 117, 134, 135, 142, 154, 160, 162, 167, 217

Nervous system, 66, 106, 202, 207, 247, 258

Neurotransmitter, 76–77, 108

New thinking, 23–29

Nitrogen, 81, 94

Non–genetically modified, 88

Nutrients, 12, 17, 24, 28, 30–31, 38, 61, 64–65, 66, 68, 71, 72, 84, 87, 92, 95, 99–100, 101, 103, 116, 122, 124, 145, 147, 150, 151, 155, 158, 169, 170, 174, 220, 221

Nutrition, 9, 10, 12–14, 16–41, 43–45, 50–51, 53–57, 59–62, 64–136, 138, 140–142, 147–152, 156–164, 166–191, 216–218, 220–222, 227–245

Nutritional composition, 17, 18, 169–174

O

Oat bran, 69, 154.
In recipes: 231

Oat milk, 40, 60, 86, 121, 154, 162

Oats, 37, 39, 40, 60, 68, 69, 70, 71, 74, 87, 92, 95, 130, 147, 154, 170, 218, 220.
In recipes: 227, 228, 230, 239, 243, 245

Obesity, 10, 12, 27, 97, 101, 114, 119–120, 122–123, 124, 133

Old thinking, 23–29, 181

Oleic acid, 102

Olive oil, 17, 26, 39, 40, 55, 95, 96, 97, 103, 114, 117, 134, 135, 140, 141, 146, 148, 149, 150, 154, 161, 162, 167, 169, 171, 172, 186, 187, 188, 190, 218, 219, 227.
In recipes: 229, 230, 232, 233, 234, 235, 236, 237, 238, 239, 240, 241, 242

Olives, 103, 117, 155, 167

Omega-3, 85, 97, 100, 104, 105–112, 113, 114, 115, 116, 117, 121, 149, 150, 167, 221.
See also polyunsaturated fats.

Omega-6, 27, 96, 97–98, 100, 104, 106, 110, 111, 112–115, 116, 117, 149, 150, 167, 221.
See also polyunsaturated fats.

Omega-9, 100, 102–104, 110, 116, 117.
See also monounsaturated fats.

Orange roughy, 85, 111

Organic, 38, 39, 40, 43–45, 84, 85, 86, 87, 88, 90, 92, 94, 120, 121, 147, 152, 153, 221

Osteoarthritis, 49, 54, 97, 99, 105, 113, 114, 124

Osteoporosis, 35, 49, 125, 128, 129–130

Ostrich, 86, 154, 167.
In recipes: 236

Oxidation level, 20

Oxidize, 103

P

Palm kernel oils, 40

Pancreas, 71, 72

Pancreatitis, 124

Partially hydrogenated, 27, 31, 42, 55, 91, 92, 98, 100, 101, 117, 120, 134, 149, 152, 167, 217, 221, 224

Pecans, 40, 103, 117

Perceived exertion, 206, 207

Personal trainer, 196, 208, 214

pH levels, 20, 34–41, 93, 125, 129, 204

Phosphate, 39, 130, 131

Phosphoric acid, 36, 37, 39, 119, 130, 131

Phytochemicals, 19, 22, 66, 68

Pilates, 201

Pistachios, 103, 117

Polyunsaturated fats, 27, 100, 103, 104–115, 149, 150. *See also* omega-3, omega-6.

Pork, 19, 40, 86, 154, 167

Postpartum depression, 108

Posture alignment, 199–200, 201, 203, 204–205, 207, 208–209, 210, 211, 218, 246, 251, 258, 281

Potassium, 35, 79, 125, 170

Poultry, 26, 40, 43, 70, 74, 81, 84, 86, 92, 95, 154, 162, 167, 186.
In recipes: 229, 232, 235, 236, 237, 238, 239, 240, 241

Processed foods, 13, 31, 35, 39, 40, 43, 66, 67, 68, 73, 78, 80, 88, 96, 97, 100, 103, 104, 113, 115, 117, 122–123, 130, 131, 149, 152

Processed snacks, *see* processed foods.

Prostaglandins, 106, 112, 113

Protein, 12, 17, 18, 19–20, 22, 26, 28, 35, 38–39, 60, 61, 64–65, 67, 72, 73, 74, 81–94, 100, 101, 115, 129–130, 131, 151, 154, 163, 166, 167, 169–174, 180, 218, 221

Protein bars (or energy bars), 90–91, 134, 150.
In recipes: 230

Protein metabolism, 93

Protein supplements, 87–89

Protein types, 81–82, 83–91, 94, 154, 167, 221

Pumpkin, 40, 153

Pumpkin seed oil, 105, 110, 112, 113, 167, 221

Pumpkin seeds, 40, 105, 110, 113, 117, 131, 154, 221

Purified water, 40, 126

Q

Quadriceps, 252, 253, 254, 255, 256, 258, 259, 260, 261, 276, 279

Quality protein, 12, 18, 26, 82, 83, 87, 89, 90, 92, 175, 218, 221

Quantity of food, 23, 24, 25, 32, 60, 75, 81, 93, 94, 121, 123, 144, 158, 162–164, 188, 204–205

Quick-pick food list, 166–167, 168

R

Raisins, 40, 70, 74, 75, 87, 130, 154, 166, 170.
In recipes: 231, 233, 244

Raspberries, 40, 70, 131, 154, 166

Raw nuts, 70, 97, 113, 114, 117, 154, 155

Recipes, 227–245

Apple crisp, 245

Baked eggplant, 241

Black bean mango salad, 232

Buffalo/turkey meatloaf, 239

Caesar salad dressing, 234

Carrot cake, 244

Cherry chicken salad, 232

Chicken and vegetable pizza, 240

CJ's big salad, 233

CJ's granola, 228

CJ's oatmeal on-the-run, 227

CJ's smoothie, 231

Cookies that "rock," 243

Energized bars, 230

Fast chicken noodle soup, 235

Flax bran muffins, 231

Greek tomato salad, 242

Oatmeal pancakes, 230

Ostrich soup, 236

Roasted sweet potato wedges, 242

Salmon or tuna patties, 240

Salmon salad, 233

Salmon teriyaki, 241

Scrambled eggs, 229

So simple salad dressing, 234

Sweet potato minestrone, 237

Taco seasoning, 245

White chicken chili, 238

Recovery phase, 207, 209, 213, 258, 284

Red meat, 40, 86, 113

Refined carbohydrates, 13, 26, 64, 66, 68, 70, 71, 73, 74, 75–77, 78, 82, 94, 115, 117, 133, 134, 147, 160, 161, 170, 172

Releasing hormone, 24, 72, 100, 123, 163

Repetitions, 208–209, 247

Reproductive system, 106

Resistance, 207, 208, 209, 211, 258

Rest and recovery, 39, 47, 48–50, 51, 53, 140, 192, 213, 218, 222, 258, 284

Restaurants, 12, 115, 178, 180, 185–187

Resting metabolic rate, 25

Restricting calories, 10, 17, 18, 25–26, 27, 29, 30–31, 33, 144, 156, 158, 162–164

Reverse osmosis, 126

Rib cage, 246, 251, 264, 269, 276

Rice milk, 40, 60, 82, 86, 121, 154

Roadblocks, 142, 143, 177

Root vegetables, 69

Rubber tubing, 201, 208, 210, 280

S

Safflower, 40, 103, 112, 113, 115, 117, 154

Salmon, 17, 82, 85, 92, 105, 110, 111, 128, 130, 141, 146, 154, 167, 187, 188, 189, 190. **In recipes:** 233, 240, 241

Satiety, 96, 218

Saturated fats, 27, 84, 86, 96, 97, 100, 101–102, 106, 113, 116, 117, 149, 150, 167, 172, 221

Sea salt, 39, 40, 131, 155. **In recipes:** 228, 229, 231, 233, 235, 236, 237, 238, 239, 241, 242, 243, 244, 245

Sea vegetables, 30, 37, 39, 40, 71, 131, 158, 222

Seeds, 15, 39, 40, 69, 70, 97, 101, 103, 104, 105, 109, 110, 112, 113, 114, 115, 117, 131, 154, 218, 221. **In recipes:** 228

Serotonin, 76, 77, 108

Serving sizes, 59, 110, 117, 145, 148–149, 152, 164, 166, 168

Sesame oil, 40, 113, 154, 167, 221

Seven Countries Study, 96

Shortening, 100, 117, 167

Shoulders, 195, 196, 200, 246, 248, 251, 252, 253, 254, 255, 256, 257, 259, 260, 261, 262, 263, 264, 265, 267, 268, 270, 271, 272, 275, 276, 277, 278, 279, 280, 286

Sirloin, 19, 154

Skiing, 201, 204, 205, 224, 264

Sleep, 23, 24, 33, 38, 39, 40, 47, 48, 49, 50, 51, 53, 54, 70, 76, 131, 140, 144, 145, 146, 179, 180, 194, 199, 212, 213, 218, 222, 289

Sleep apnea, 54

Smoothies, 74, 78, 88, 89, 90, 102, 109, 110, 114, 117, 118, 135, 141, 142, 146, 156, 173, 189, 190, 219. **In recipes:** 231

Snacks, 17, 18, 19, 23, 24, 55, 88, 89, 90, 97, 98, 103, 114, 117, 123, 134, 135, 136, 140, 141, 146, 157, 163, 164, 169, 170, 173, 174, 179, 181, 185, 186, 188, 189, 190, 191, 212, 289.
In recipes: 228, 230–231

Soda pop, 18, 34, 35, 36, 37, 40, 68, 77, 80, 119–120, 123, 125, 127, 130, 131, 134, 161, 171, 172, 173, 184, 187

Sodium, 35, 125, 153, 155

Soluble fiber, 69

Soy burgers, 92

Soy chicken, 92

Soy milk, 40, 60, 74, 82, 83, 86, 87, 121, 128, 146, 154, 158, 160, 164, 167, 170, 188, 189.
In recipes: 227, 230, 231, 240

Soy protein isolate, 87

Soybean oil, 96, 97, 98, 112, 113, 115, 117

Soybeans, 40, 71, 74, 87, 92, 110, 113, 115, 117, 130, 167

Speed of movement, 208, 209

Spirituality, 179, 180

Splenda, 40

Splits, 208, 213, 283, 284

Spring water, 126, 142, 218, 220

Stability and balance, 129, 131, 132, 139, 198, 201, 202, 203, 207, 208, 209, 219, 251, 258

Stair climbers, 286

Starchy carbohydrates, 76, 77, 220

Starvation, 7, 23, 68, 156

Stevia plant, 77

Stevia Plus™, 77–78, 155, 166.
In recipes: 228, 231, 243, 244

Storing, 110, 113

Strength training, 15, 42, 129, 131, 162, 195, 197, 198, 199, 200, 201, 202, 207–209, 210, 212, 213, 222, 258–272, 282, 283, 284, 285, 286, 290

Strength training phase, 207–209, 258

Stress, 16, 25, 29, 35, 36, 37, 38, 39, 40, 41, 42, 48, 50, 53, 76, 93, 120, 130, 131, 162, 163, 168, 176, 180, 181, 188, 194, 199, 204, 205, 207, 209, 215, 222, 258, 273

Stretching, 197, 199, 201, 202, 209–210, 211, 213, 222, 247, 248, 273–280, 282, 283, 284, 285

Sucrolose, 150

Sugar, 26, 35, 39, 40, 42, 66, 67, 68, 71, 73, 74, 75, 77, 78, 80, 119, 122, 123, 130, 134, 148, 150, 151, 155, 160, 165, 166, 170, 175, 217.
In recipes: 231, 243, 244, 245

Sumo wrestler, 23, 24, 72, 76, 156, 157

Sunflower (seeds, oil), 103, 112, 113, 114, 117, 154, 167, 221.
In recipes: 228

Supplements, 10, 16, 27, 28, 29, 87–89, 221

Swimming, 52, 201, 204, 205, 213, 224

Swissball, 209, 211

Swordfish, 85, 111

T

Tai chi, 201

Talk test, 206, 207

Taurine, 124

Tea, 39, 40, 120–121, 127, 131, 138, 160, 221, 222

Tempeh, 40, 167

Testimonials, 10, 15, 17, 20, 29, 42, 44, 51, 52, 58, 60, 91, 107, 123, 131, 132, 143, 165, 168, 174, 183, 185, 201, 215, 217, 225

Testosterone, 204, 205, 207

Thanksgiving, 76, 163

Thermogenesis, 112

Thermogenic, 124

Thermoregulation, 27

Three-hour rule, the, 156–157, 163, 222

Tofu, 37, 81, 130, 154, 167

Training specificity, 202, 205

Trans-fatty acids, 27, 31, 32, 96–97, 98, 99, 100–101, 106, 114, 116, 117, 119, 120, 134, 147, 148, 149, 150, 167, 186, 217, 221

Treadmill, 197, 286

Tropical oils, 117

Trout, 85, 105, 111

Tuna, 70, 85, 105, 111, 130, 141, 146, 154, 167, 171, 184, 185, 186, 189.
In recipes: 233, 240

Turkey, 40, 86, 154, 161, 167, 189.
In recipes: 229, 237, 239, 241

Type 2 diabetes, 12, 24, 27, 32, 97, 99, 106, 107, 120, 123, 125, 133, 195

U

Ulcers, 124

Unrefined, 26, 27, 64, 68, 71, 73, 77, 79, 92, 103, 113, 114, 117, 149, 154, 155

Upward dog, 210, 257, 278, 279, 283, 284

USDA Food Pyramid, 59–61

V

Vegetable oils, 100, 112

Venison, 55, 86, 154, 167

Vitamin D, 130–131, 180

Vitamins, 13, 19, 20, 22, 26, 27, 66, 67, 68, 74, 81, 84, 99, 101, 122, 130–131, 170, 171, 180, 218, 220, 221, 222

W

Waistline, 25, 26, 27, 33, 64, 185, 186, 187, 195

Walking, 42, 52, 131, 140, 162, 197, 198, 199, 201, 202, 203, 204, 205, 213, 216, 218, 224, 247, 251, 286

Walnuts, 35, 40, 70, 74, 87, 105, 110, 114, 117, 141, 146, 154, 164, 167, 170, 189, 218, 221.
In recipes: 231, 232, 243, 244

Water-insoluble fiber, 69

Water-soluble fiber, 69

Weight loss, 8, 9, 14, 15, 16–22, 23, 25, 26, 29, 30–31, 32, 42, 49, 52, 54–55, 67, 95, 96, 99, 100, 102, 105–106, 112–113, 144–145, 156–157, 158–168, 176, 182, 195–196, 198–199, 204–205, 217, 219–222

Wheat grass, 30, 40, 71, 122, 130, 138, 140, 141, 153, 158, 159, 160, 215, 219, 221, 222

Whey, 87, 88, 154, 167.
In recipes: 230, 231, 243

Whey protein isolate, 87

White bread, 68, 70, 71, 73, 74, 92, 134, 142, 147, 160, 161, 170, 171

White fat, 112

Whole grains, 12, 19, 39, 44, 59, 68, 69, 70, 71, 77, 154, 218, 220, 221

Whole-grain bread, 18, 70, 71, 73, 77, 78, 81, 82, 87, 92, 103, 134, 135, 142, 147, 154, 161, 166, 189, 190

World Health Organization, 114

Y

Yoga, 52, 131, 140, 162, 165, 179, 197, 198, 200, 201, 202, 210, 211, 286

Yogurt, 17, 40, 73, 74, 86, 109, 110, 111, 114, 142, 154, 167, 172, 188, 190, 191, 219

Yolk, 84, 85, 117

Z

Zinc, 87

On Target Living— **PERSONAL NOTES**

On Target Living— **PERSONAL NOTES**

On Target Living— **PERSONAL NOTES**

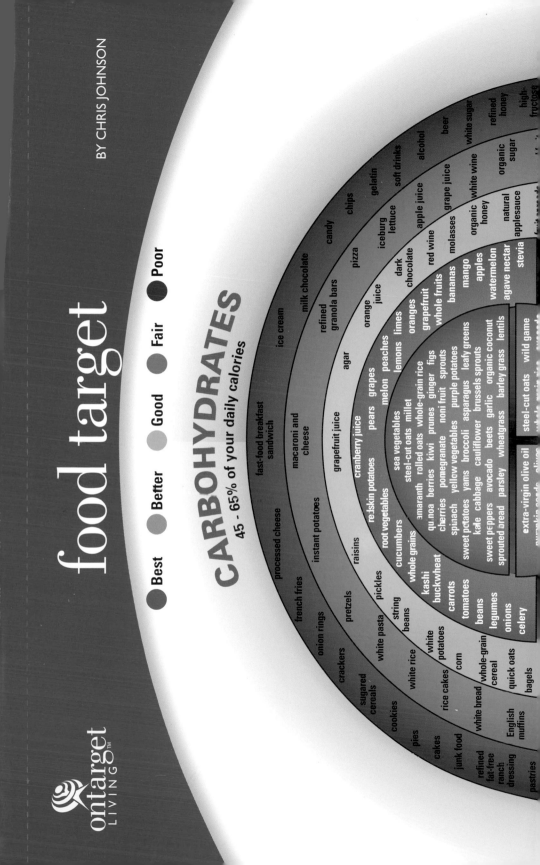

food target

BY CHRIS JOHNSON

ontarget
LIVING™

● Best ● Better ● Good ● Fair ● Poor

CARBOHYDRATES
45 - 65% of your daily calories

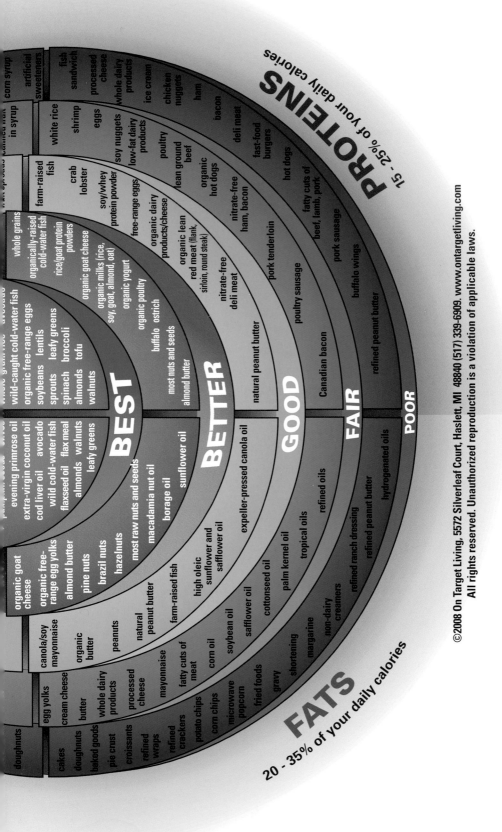

PROTEINS
15 - 25% of your daily calories

FATS
20 - 35% of your daily calories

BEST

BETTER

GOOD

FAIR

POOR

Proteins — BEST:
evening primrose oil, extra-virgin coconut oil, cod liver oil, wild cold-water fish, flaxseed oil, flax meal, almonds, walnuts, leafy greens, wild-caught cold-water fish, organic free-range eggs, soybeans, lentils, sprouts, leafy greens, spinach, broccoli, almonds, tofu, walnuts, whole grains, organically-raised cold-water fish, rice/goat protein powders, organic goat cheese, organic milks (rice, soy, goat, almond, oat), soy/whey protein powder, free-range eggs, organic dairy products/cheese, organic yogurt, organic poultry, buffalo, ostrich, most nuts and seeds, almond butter, farm-raised fish, shrimp, crab, lobster, eggs, soy nuggets, low-fat dairy products, poultry, lean ground beef, organic hot dogs, nitrate-free ham, bacon, farm-raised fish, white rice, fish sandwich, processed cheese, whole dairy products, ice cream, chicken nuggets, ham, bacon, deli meat, fast-food burgers, corn syrup, artificial sweeteners

Proteins — BETTER / GOOD:
organic lean red meat (flank, sirloin, round steak), nitrate-free deli meat, pork tenderloin, Canadian bacon, poultry sausage, pork sausage, fatty cuts of beef, lamb, pork, hot dogs, deli meat

Proteins — FAIR / POOR:
buffalo wings, refined peanut butter

Fats — BEST:
organic goat cheese, organic free-range egg yolks, almond butter, pine nuts, brazil nuts, hazelnuts, most raw nuts and seeds, macadamia nut oil, borage oil, sunflower oil

Fats — BETTER:
high oleic sunflower and safflower oil, expeller-pressed canola oil

Fats — GOOD:
natural peanut butter, safflower oil, cottonseed oil, soybean oil, corn oil, high oleic sunflower and safflower oil

Fats — FAIR:
palm kernel oil, tropical oils, refined oils

Fats — POOR:
canola/soy mayonnaise, organic butter, whole dairy products, processed cheese, mayonnaise, fatty cuts of meat, corn chips, microwave popcorn, potato chips, fried foods, gravy, shortening, margarine, non-dairy creamers, refined ranch dressing, refined peanut butter, hydrogenated oils

doughnuts, egg yolks, cream cheese, butter, whole dairy products, processed cheese, mayonnaise, refined crackers, cakes, doughnuts, baked goods, pie crust, croissants, refined wraps

©2008 On Target Living, 5572 Silverleaf Court, Haslett, MI 48840 (517) 339-6909. www.ontargetliving.com
All rights reserved. Unauthorized reproduction is a violation of applicable laws.